Tackling HIV-Related Stigma and Discrimination in South Asia

Tackling HIV-Related Stigma and Discrimination in South Asia

Anne Stangl, Dara Carr, Laura Brady, Traci Eckhaus,
Mariam Claeson, and Laura Nyblade

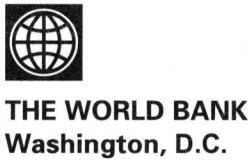

THE WORLD BANK
Washington, D.C.

© 2010 The International Bank for Reconstruction and Development / The World Bank
1818 H Street NW
Washington DC 20433
Telephone: 202-473-1000
Internet: www.worldbank.org
E-mail: feedback@worldbank.org

1 2 3 4 13 12 11 10

This volume is a product of the staff of the International Bank for Reconstruction and Development / The World Bank. The findings, interpretations, and conclusions expressed in this volume do not necessarily reflect the views of the Executive Directors of The World Bank or the governments they represent.

The World Bank does not guarantee the accuracy of the data included in this work. The boundaries, colors, denominations, and other information shown on any map in this work do not imply any judgement on the part of The World Bank concerning the legal status of any territory or the endorsement or acceptance of such boundaries.

Rights and Permissions
The material in this publication is copyrighted. Copying and/or transmitting portions or all of this work without permission may be a violation of applicable law. The International Bank for Reconstruction and Development / The World Bank encourages dissemination of its work and will normally grant permission to reproduce portions of the work promptly.

For permission to photocopy or reprint any part of this work, please send a request with complete information to the Copyright Clearance Center Inc., 222 Rosewood Drive, Danvers, MA 01923, USA; telephone: 978-750-8400; fax: 978-750-4470; Internet: www.copyright.com.

All other queries on rights and licenses, including subsidiary rights, should be addressed to the Office of the Publisher, The World Bank, 1818 H Street NW, Washington, DC 20433, USA; fax: 202-522-2422; e-mail: pubrights@worldbank.org

ISBN: 978-0-8213-8449-7
eISBN: 978-0-8213-8451-0
DOI: 10.1596/978-0-8213-8449-7

Library of Congress Cataloging-in-Publication Data
Tackling HIV-related stigma and discrimination in South Asia / Anne Stangl ... [et al.].
    p. ; cm.
Includes bibliographical references and index.
ISBN 978-0-8213-8449-7 — ISBN 978-0-8213-8451-0 (electronic)
1. AIDS (Disease)—South Asia. 2. Stigma (Social psychology)—South Asia. I. Stang, Anne. II. World Bank.
[DNLM: 1. HIV Infections—psychology—Afghanistan. 2. HIV Infections—psychology—Asia, Western. 3. Health Education—standards—Afghanistan. 4. Health Education—standards—Asia, Western. 5. Health Knowledge, Attitudes, Practice—Afghanistan. 6. Health Knowledge, Attitudes, Practice—Asia, Western. 7. Health Promotion—standards—Afghanistan. 8. Health Promotion—standards—Asia, Western. 9. International Cooperation—Afghanistan. 10. International Cooperation—Asia, Western. 11. Prejudice—Afghanistan. 12. Prejudice—Asia, Western. WC 503.7 T118 2010]
RA643.86.S67T33 2010
362.196'979200954—dc22
                                                                                    2010022090

Cover photo: Shehab Uddin/Drik/Majority World
The cover photo shows Rupali and Mithu, who work as community health workers for the Society for Positive Atmosphere and Related Support to HIV/AIDS (SPARSHA) to reduce HIV-related stigma in the villages of West Bengal. They live openly with HIV.
Cover design: Naylor Design, Washington, DC

Contents

Boxes

Figure

Tables

Preface

In its 2008 round, Tackling HIV and AIDS Stigma and Discrimination, the South Asia Region Development Marketplace[1] (SARDM) supported 26 implementers from six countries to pilot innovative interventions over a 12- to 18-month period. Total grant support was US$1.04 million, with a maximum grant size of US$40,000. In making these grants, SARDM focused on field innovators. After consulting with stakeholders, including marginalized populations most affected by stigma, SARDM offered relatively small grant amounts to ensure that these groups and community organizations would be able to compete with larger groups. The response to the initial call for proposals was immense, with almost a thousand submissions from Afghanistan, Bangladesh, Bhutan, India, Nepal, Pakistan, and Sri Lanka.

The findings in this report are based on project monitoring and evaluation data collected by SARDM implementers and six case studies conducted by the International Center for Research on Women (ICRW). No one formula can capture the diversity and ingenuity reflected in this body of work. However, the findings do suggest some broad crosscutting principles as well as programmatic lessons associated with specific approaches.

In terms of broad lessons and principles, the experiences of SARDM implementers suggest the following:

- *Community organizations can achieve a great deal for relatively little investment.* The 26 SARDM implementers reached 96,264 people, trained 4,905 people, led to 504 news articles, and developed 426 products such as training curricula; information, education, and communication materials; documentaries; and plays. Overall, the results suggest a high return on investment.
- *Development Marketplace grants seeded considerable innovation.* Project approaches reflected enormous creativity, ranging from beauty pageants to restaurants run by sex workers. The grants led to new alliances, such as those between panchayat (municipal government) leaders and community organizations. They also led to some unlikely partnerships, such as sex workers and the police, and new insights on engaging religious leaders.
- *The most effective projects required substantial up-front planning and effort.* Regardless of the implementer's particular approach or population served, the most promising projects invested considerable time and effort in engaging gatekeepers, conducting formative research on different audiences, training, forming new partnerships, and other activities.
- *The most promising work uses multiple strategies and stakeholders to address stigma.* Even where projects initially appeared to be single-focus interventions (for example, theater), successful implementation required a range of other activities, such as training, engaging with policy makers, and cultivating media relations.
- *Effective efforts are led by or continuously engage marginalized communities.* Involving marginalized communities is essential for strengthening capacity, ensuring appropriate messaging, and maximizing results. Strategies that foster some interaction between marginalized communities and the public can be powerful in inspiring change. Products such as films or plays that marginalized communities developed or helped inform are likely to be more compelling to audiences.

In addition to these broad lessons, a number of program lessons emerged in connection with specific intervention approaches. For most SARDM implementers, buy-in from government and opinion leaders was essential for carrying out interventions on sensitive issues. Many implementers inspired the support of these groups by appealing to positive values such as compassion and by publicly rewarding people whose attitudes and behaviors are already respectful and supportive of marginalized populations.

Government support greatly extends the reach of the work of community organizations and helps broker new alliances, such as those with religious leaders.

Capacity strengthening was an important element of implementation. Addressing self-stigma (the internalization of society's negative attitudes) is often a precondition for the participation of marginalized populations in activities. Linking communities with support options is critical, both for addressing self-stigma and for encouraging service use. In another form of capacity strengthening, implementing organizations benefited by partnering with professionals or other organizations with specialized expertise. Finally, providing economic opportunities to beneficiaries was found to reduce stigma on multiple fronts, thus strengthening capacity. These efforts can be even more effective if coupled with stigma reduction programming and links to support and other services. However, community organizations may find formal sector employment approaches challenging, especially where jobs are scarce.

Cultural and media approaches were an effective means of broaching sensitive topics and addressing drivers of stigma, such as cultural attitudes regarding sexuality. Plays, films, and other products tended to be more effective when rooted in real-life experiences. Recruiting people from marginalized communities proved crucial but could be difficult, especially if public disclosure was involved. Links to networks and groups for support can facilitate safe participation. Additionally, effective efforts to involve people from marginalized communities require skill and experience so as not to unintentionally reinforce harmful stereotypes.

Technical assistance to implementers, provided through ICRW, included stigma reduction programming, messaging, and monitoring and evaluation. SARDM implementers collected formative and monitoring data to strengthen implementation, report outcomes, and document lessons. Upfront training combined with a mix of proactive and on-demand technical assistance best met the needs of implementers, who had greatly varying levels of experience. For a number of implementers, a next step would be more intensive technical support to undertake quantitative evaluation of their programs' effect.

The experiences of SARDM implementers provide a strong foundation on which to build stigma reduction efforts in the region (see table P.1).

To spur further innovation and scale, recommendations include the following:

• Promote intensified government support for a scaled-up response to stigma and discrimination.

Table P.1   Highlights from Experiences of 26 SARDM Implementers

Types of implementers	Organizations
Implementers that developed new training, cultural, or media products	• Afghan Family Guidance Association (Afghanistan) • Afghan Help and Training Program (Afghanistan) • Concern Worldwide (Afghanistan) • Drik Picture Library (Bangladesh) • JOBS Trust (Bangladesh) • Development Initiative (India) • ISTV Network (India) • Lotus Integrated AIDS Awareness Sangam (India) • Nalandaway Foundation (India) • Sai Paranjpye Films (India) • Society for Positive Atmosphere and Related Support to HIV/AIDS (India) • The Communication Hub (India) • Voluntary Health Association of Tripura (India) • We Care Social Service Society (India) • Federation of Sexual and Gender Minorities Nepal • Himalayan Association against STI-AIDS (Nepal) • New Light AIDS Control Society (Pakistan) • Lanka+ (Sri Lanka)
Implementers that established buy-in and support from groups that rarely engage in stigma reduction programs, such as police, local policy makers, and religious leaders	• Afghan Family Guidance Association (Afghanistan) • Afghan Help and Training Program (Afghanistan) • Concern Worldwide (Afghanistan) • Ashodaya Samithi (India) • Lotus Integrated AIDS Awareness Sangam (India) • Saral (India) • Voluntary Health Association of Tripura (India)
Implementers that staged events and programs reaching thousands of viewers	• Afghan Help and Training Program (Afghanistan) • Ashodaya Samithi (India) • Development Initiative (India) • ISTV Network (India) • Lotus Integrated AIDS Awareness Sangam (India) • Sai Paranjpye Films (India) • Federation of Sexual and Gender Minorities Nepal • Pakistan Press Foundation (Pakistan) • Alliance Lanka (Sri Lanka)
Implementers that challenged stigma in institutional settings, such as health care and universities	• Afghan Family Guidance Association (Afghanistan) • Concern Worldwide (Afghanistan) • Ashodaya Samithi (India) • Saral (India) • National NGOs Network Group against AIDS–Nepal • New Light AIDS Control Society (Pakistan) • Integrated Health Services (Pakistan)

(continued)

Table P.1   Highlights from Experiences of 26 SARDM Implementers *(continued)*

Types of implementers	*Organizations*
Implementers that generated new nonstigmatizing media articles	• Nari Unnayan Shakti (Bangladesh) • Swathi Mahila Sangha, Vijaya Mahila Sangha, Jyothi Mahila Sangha, Swasti Health Resource Center (India) • The Communication Hub (India) • Voluntary Health Association of Tripura (India) • New Light AIDS Control Society (Pakistan) • Pakistan Press Foundation (Pakistan)
Implementers that used a cascading training-of-trainers approach to extend reach and influence	• Afghan Family Guidance Association (Afghanistan) • Afghan Help and Training Program (Afghanistan) • National NGOs Network Group against AIDS–Nepal • New Light AIDS Control Society (Pakistan)
Implementers that worked with vulnerable populations such as men who have sex with men, injecting drug users, sex workers, and people living with HIV	• Afghan Family Guidance Association (Afghanistan) • Concern Worldwide (Afghanistan) • JOBS Trust (Bangladesh) • Ashodaya Samithi (India) • Lotus Integrated AIDS Awareness Sangam (India) • Sai Paranjpye Films (India) • Saral (India) • Society for Positive Atmosphere and Related Support to HIV/AIDS (India) • The Communication Hub (India) • Voluntary Health Association of Tripura (India) • We Care Social Service Society (India) • Federation of Sexual and Gender Minorities Nepal • Himalayan Association against STI-AIDS (Nepal) • National NGOs Network Group against AIDS–Nepal • New Light AIDS Control Society (Pakistan) • Alliance Lanka (Sri Lanka) • Lanka+ (Sri Lanka)
Implementers that generated income to support project activities or program beneficiaries	• JOBS Trust (Bangladesh) • Saral (India) • Lanka+ (Sri Lanka)
Implementers that mobilized additional donor funds for activities related to their SARDM projects	• Nalandaway Foundation (India) • Society for Positive Atmosphere and Related Support to HIV/AIDS (India) • Federation of Sexual and Gender Minorities Nepal • Lanka+ (Sri Lanka)
Implementers that inspired the development of new networks or support organizations	• Concern Worldwide (Afghanistan) • Nari Unnayan Shakti (Bangladesh) • Ashodaya Samithi (India) • National NGOs Network Group against AIDS–Nepal • Alliance Lanka (Sri Lanka)

Source: Authors' compilation.

- Promote government adoption of stigma reduction efforts in health care.
- Encourage replication of promising SARDM approaches through organization-to-organization knowledge transfer.
- Promote use of multipronged programming strategies for increased effectiveness.
- Leverage cultural and media efforts of SARDM implementers to maximize reach and results.
- Further sharpen and refine tools that religious leaders can use to discourage stigma and discrimination and to promote tolerance.
- Foster stronger private sector engagement for greater economic opportunity among marginalized populations.
- Ensure that an expanded response to stigma and discrimination includes economic opportunities for marginalized populations.
- Support implementers in strengthening their capacity to expand.

Note

1. The South Asia Region Development Marketplace partnership is sponsored by the World Bank Group, including the International Finance Corporation; the government of Norway; the Joint United Nations Programme on HIV/AIDS; the Swedish International Development Cooperation Agency; the United Nations Children's Fund; and the United Nations Development Programme.

Acknowledgments

A team from the International Center for Research on Women wrote this report. The team comprised Anne Stangl, Dara Carr, Laura Brady, Traci Eckhaus, and Laura Nyblade, with contributions from Mariam Claeson (World Bank). Margo Young and Sandy Won (International Center for Research on Women) and Phoebe Folger (World Bank) provided editorial support.

The content of the report reflects the dedicated work of the 26 South Asia Region Development Marketplace (SARDM) implementing organizations and their partner organizations and would not have been possible without the efforts and successes of the following groups:

Afghan Family Guidance Association; Afghan Help and Training Program; Alliance Lanka; Ashodaya Samithi; Concern Worldwide and Action Aid; Development Initiative; Drik Picture Library; Federation of Sexual and Gender Minorities Nepal; Himalayan Association against STI-AIDS; Integrated Health Services; ISTV Network with the Institute of Social Work and Research; JOBS Trust; Lanka+; Lotus Integrated AIDS Awareness Sangam; Nalandaway Foundation; Nari Unnayan Shakti; National NGOs Network Group against AIDS–Nepal; New Light AIDS Control Society; Pakistan Press Foundation; Sai Paranjpye Films; Saral and Aadhar; Society for Positive Atmosphere and Related Support to

HIV/AIDS with MAKE ART/STOP AIDS and the National Institute of Cholera and Enteric Diseases; Swathi Mahila Sangha, Vijaya Mahila Sangha, Jyothi Mahila Sangha, and Swasti Health Resource Centre; The Communication Hub and the Network of Maharashtra People Living with HIV; Voluntary Health Association of Tripura; and We Care Social Service Society.

The South Asia Region Development Marketplace was coordinated by Mariam Claeson and the team at the World Bank, including Phoebe Folger, Ruby Singh, Rosalind Rajan, Tanya Ringland, Sunita Vanjani, Shirin Jahangeer, Hasib Karimzada, Huma Ali Waheed, Anne Bossuyt, Kumari Navaratne, Sundar Gopalan, Ghulam Dastagir Sayed, Ayesha Ahmad, Shanaz Kazi, Nastu Sharma, Kerima Thilakasena, Jaya Karki, Keiko Nagai, and Nandiny Kesavaswamy. The SARDM on stigma received generous financial support from the SARDM 2008 partnership, sponsored by the World Bank Group including the International Finance Corporation, the Government of Norway, the Joint United Nations Programme on HIV/AIDS, the Swedish International Development Cooperation Agency, the United Nations Children's Fund, and the United Nations Development Programme.

The team gratefully acknowledges the generous support of the Government of the Netherlands through the Bank-Netherlands Partnership Program for this publication.

The national AIDS programs of Afghanistan, Bangladesh, Bhutan, India, Nepal, Pakistan, and Sri Lanka supported the South Asia Region Development Marketplace from the launch through implementation to the regional knowledge forum in March 2010, when the lessons learned were disseminated.

Contributors

Anne Stangl is a behavioral scientist and stigma specialist at the International Center for Research on Women. She has extensive experience conducting qualitative and quantitative research related to HIV stigma; developing tools to measure stigma; and providing program and policy guidance to agencies and organizations at the global, national, and community levels. She is the secretariat coordinator of a global HIV stigma reduction network of researchers, implementers, advocates, HIV-affected populations, and development partners to foster knowledge sharing and enhanced coordination around stigma reduction. Dr. Stangl holds a PhD in public health from Tulane University.

Dara Carr is an independent consultant based in Portland, Oregon. She is an analyst and writer specializing in gender, HIV, and reproductive health. Her experience includes working with donors, governments, and civil society organizations worldwide to improve public health policies and programs. She previously worked at the Population Reference Bureau, World Bank, and Demographic and Health Surveys program.

Laura Brady is a program associate at the International Center for Research on Women (ICRW). She plays critical coordinating, managing, and technical support roles to facilitate the center's extensive research, programming, and technical assistance work on HIV stigma around the world. Specifically, she assists with conducting literature reviews and other secondary data searches; performing quantitative and qualitative data analysis and interpretation; drafting and editing reports; and providing technical input to project development, design, and implementation. Before joining ICRW, she worked for several years in Latin America, the Caribbean, Africa, and Asia, and more recently in Tanzania and Trinidad with the CDC Global AIDS Program. She holds an MPH from the George Washington University.

Traci Eckhaus is a program assistant at the International Center for Research on Women. She works closely with the HIV and Gender Team and the Stigma, Discrimination, and Gender Team, providing financial management and administrative backstopping, literature searches, and assistance with data analysis. She holds a BA in anthropology and Spanish from Washington University in St. Louis.

Mariam Claeson, MD, MPH, is the regional program coordinator for AIDS in the South Asia Region of the World Bank since 2005. She was the coordinator of the South Asia Region Development Marketplace 2008 partnership, which supported the innovations to tackle HIV-related stigma and discrimination that are summarized in this report. She has contributed to the analysis of the dynamics of the HIV epidemic in South Asia in several publications and is the team leader for World Bank support to the third National AIDS Control Project in India.

Laura Nyblade is the director of stigma, discrimination, and gender at the International Center for Research on Women. She has more than 15 years of experience in HIV research, program design, and evaluation. She is a global expert on HIV stigma and is a co-creator of *Challenging HIV-Stigma: Toolkit for Action*, now translated into seven languages and used around the world. In addition to focusing on translational research, Dr. Nyblade provides technical guidance on stigma reduction policy and programming to international agencies, including the Joint United Nations Programme on HIV/AIDS, the U.K. Department for International Development, and the World Bank. She holds a PhD in demography from the University of Pennsylvania.

Abbreviations

ACT	Advocacy by Cultural Teams
AFGA	Afghan Family Guidance Association
AHTP	Afghan Help and Training Program
AIDS	acquired immunodeficiency syndrome
AMT	Aadhar Mahila Trust (India)
ART	antiretroviral therapy
BCC	behavior change communication
BDS	Blue Diamond Society (Nepal)
BSF	Border Security Force (India)
CD	compact disc
CFAR	Centre for Advocacy and Research (India)
CHW	community health worker
CSO	civil society organization
DACC	District AIDS Coordination Committee (Nepal)
DVD	digital video disc
FSGMN	Federation of Sexual and Gender Minorities Nepal
HASTI-AIDS	Himalayan Association against STI-AIDS (Nepal)
HIV	human immunodeficiency virus
HNI-TPO	HealthNet International and the Transcultural Psycho-social Organisation
ICRW	International Center for Research on Women

IDU	injecting drug user
IEC	information, education, and communication
IHS	Integrated Health Services (Pakistan)
INP+	Indian Network for People Living with HIV/AIDS
IV	intravenous
JACK	Just Afghan Capacity and Knowledge
JOBS	Job Opportunity and Business Support (Bangladesh)
LGBTI	lesbian, gay, bisexual, transgender, and intersex
M&E	monitoring and evaluation
MOU	memorandum of understanding
MSM	men who have sex with men
NACO	National AIDS Control Organisation (India)
NACP	National AIDS Control Program (Afghanistan)
NANGAN	National NGOs Network Group against AIDS–Nepal
NGO	nongovernmental organization
NLACS	New Light AIDS Control Society (Pakistan)
NMP+	Network of Maharashtra People with HIV (India)
NUS	Nari Unnayan Shakti (Bangladesh)
POET	Participatory Organization for Empowerment of Transgender (Pakistan)
PPF	Pakistan Press Foundation
SARDM	South Asia Region Development Marketplace
SEEDS	Sarvodaya Economic Enterprise Development Services (Sri Lanka)
SMS	Swathi Mahila Sangha (India)
SPARSHA	Society for Positive Atmosphere and Related Support to HIV/AIDS
STI	sexually transmitted infection
TCH	The Communication Hub (India)
TOT	training-of-trainers
TV	television
UNAIDS	Joint United Nations Programme on HIV/AIDS
UNICEF	United Nations Children's Fund
UNMAAI	United Network of MSM Advocacy and AIDS Initiatives (India)
UNODC	United Nations Office on Drugs and Crime
VCT	voluntary counseling and testing
VHAT	Voluntary Health Association of Tripura (India)
WDCE	workplace discipline and congenial environment

CHAPTER 1

Introduction and Background

Although HIV prevalence in South Asia is relatively low, the epidemic is growing among marginalized groups, including sex workers, injection drug users, men who have sex with men, and transgender communities (Haacker and Claeson 2009). Despite prevention and other efforts to reduce high-risk behaviors such as unprotected sex, buying and selling of sex, and injecting drug use, HIV vulnerability and risk remain high. This problem is partly due to a widespread failure to respond adequately to key social drivers of HIV: stigma and discrimination. Stigmatizing attitudes in the general population and discriminatory treatment by actors ranging from health providers to local policy makers intensify the marginalization of vulnerable groups at highest risk, driving them further from the reach of health services and much-needed prevention, treatment, care, and support. Daily harassment and abuse also cause health problems and adversely affect mental health, thereby leading to depression, social isolation, and an array of adverse socioeconomic outcomes related to HIV and AIDS.

Many people from marginalized populations do not feel as though their lives are worth taking action to protect or prolong. Muthukumar

Natesan, a leader of a community-based organization for men who have sex with men that is also working on stigma reduction, explained:

> Despite all my knowledge and years working to promote condom use, I only started using condoms consistently when I felt my existence was important. . . . [Y]ou can talk as much as you want about the need to protect oneself, you can provide as many condoms and lubricant as you want, but unless men who have sex with men feel their existence is worthwhile, they are not going to bother to protect themselves or others. . . . My existence became important and my life worth living when I received the acceptance of friends, family, neighbors, health care providers, and the community in general. Now I use condoms consistently.

Since the beginning of the HIV epidemic, public health experts and practitioners have known that stigma, discrimination, and gender inequality play an enormous role in furthering the spread of HIV. The response to these social drivers, however, remains inadequate to the scale and intensity of the challenges they pose. Despite considerable progress in recent years, many projects addressing stigma and discrimination are still small in scale or in the pilot phase. Furthermore, despite repeated recommendations for greater involvement of marginalized communities in the response to HIV, their active engagement remains scarce in most countries.

For governments and large donors, a number of issues can deter investment in work to reduce stigma. Many of the groups undertaking stigma reduction efforts, especially those led by and for marginalized populations, are relatively new and have a range of capacity needs. Although research suggests they are the best hope for community action and social change, most of these groups are currently not poised to substantially expand their work and absorb larger grant amounts. However, providing small grants may not be operationally or administratively feasible for large donors. The increasing demand by donors for quantified information on project outputs and outcomes poses additional obstacles to many community networks and groups that lack managerial and financial experience, including monitoring and evaluation skills.

The South Asia Region Development Marketplace[1] (SARDM) took an innovative and unique approach to addressing these gaps and needs through its 2008 Development Marketplace, "Tackling HIV and AIDS Stigma and Discrimination." The approach, which was informed by consultation with stakeholders, including representatives of community groups and networks of drug users, sex workers, and men having sex with men, included disbursing relatively small grant amounts; funding organizations led by and for marginalized groups; and supporting implementers in program design, monitoring, and evaluation. The call for proposals was disseminated through local media channels and in many local languages to increase outreach. Proposals could be submitted through hard copy or online in local languages, translated by the World Bank country office staff. The response to the initial call for proposals was immense, with almost 1,000 submissions from urban and rural areas in Afghanistan, Bangladesh, Bhutan, India, Nepal, Pakistan, and Sri Lanka. In 2008, the competitive grants program selected 26 implementers from six countries to pilot innovative interventions over a 12- to 18-month period. The grant funding totaled US$1.04 million, with a maximum grant size of US$40,000.

The grants program inspired these groups to implement a range of innovative and creative responses to HIV stigma and discrimination. On an organizational level, the grants also led to the development of important new skills and capabilities, positioning many of these groups for further growth and creating a base of stigma reduction expertise in the region. Technical assistance to implementers, provided through the International Center for Research on Women (ICRW), included stigma reduction programming, messaging, and monitoring and evaluation. The ICRW research team provided assistance both at specific points during the grant period and "on demand" when implementers sought support. The SARDM implementers provided midterm and final reports to the World Bank that explained their achievement of agreed-on milestones and performance targets.

Part I of this report describes key findings and lessons learned that emerged across the 26 implementers. Part II contains case studies for six of the implementers, offering a more in-depth look at the lessons and challenges of intervening against stigma and discrimination. Part III provides summaries of all 26 projects.

Note

1. The SARDM partnership is sponsored by the World Bank Group (including the International Finance Corporation), the Government of Norway, the Swedish International Development Cooperation Agency, the Joint United Nations Programme on HIV/AIDS, the United Nations Children's Fund, and the United Nations Development Programme.

Reference

Haacker, Markus, and Mariam Claeson, eds. 2009. *HIV and AIDS in South Asia: An Economic Development Risk*. Washington, DC: World Bank.

Key Findings and Lessons Learned from 26 Stigma Reduction Innovations in South Asia

CHAPTER 2

Methods

The findings in this report are based on project monitoring and evaluation data collected by implementers from the 2008 South Asia Region Development Marketplace, as reported in their midterm and final project reports, and on six case studies conducted by the International Center for Research on Women (ICRW).

Program Data

The majority of the implementers, as appropriate for their grants, collected monitoring data on project outputs (for example, numbers trained, training materials produced, articles written, plays produced) and documented outcomes linked to program activities, such as actions resulting from advocacy campaigns. Specific indicators to assess changes in stigma and discrimination over time were recommended at a regional monitoring and evaluation workshop that most implementers attended. However, few implementers could conduct quantitative surveys to gather this type of information because of both organizational capacity and budgetary constraints. Therefore, in their project reports, implementers mostly documented qualitative evaluation data based on focus group discussions and key informant interviews. Overall, 20 projects collected program monitoring data, 13 collected qualitative data, and 8 conducted surveys to inform or assess the intervention. In addition, nearly all 26 projects received a midterm visit from the joint World Bank and ICRW team.

Case Study Methodology

Six projects, described in greater detail in part II of the report, were selected as case studies to gather more in-depth information on some of the innovative strategies being implemented. Selection criteria included the potential for influence and scale, operational feasibility, and diversity of populations served. Though only six projects were included as case studies, many of their challenges, approaches taken, and lessons learned reflect those of all the implementers. Logistics and security concerns played a role in selection, and some compelling projects were eliminated because of security restrictions that limited travel to the project sites for the research team.

The research team visited each of the six case study sites at the end of the grant period in December 2009. These site visits lasted two to three days and consisted of one-on-one interviews and small-group discussions with a variety of informants, including program implementers (project directors, trainers, community mobilizers); program participants (actors, former drug users, female sex workers); and key stakeholders (media, police, government officials, community members, local government leaders). The ICRW research team conducted interviews using a semi-structured interview guide to capture key lessons about the influence of the project on individuals and communities and operational challenges in project start-up and implementation. The team also gathered relevant materials such as play scripts, communications materials, and organizational and program materials during the site visits. Field notes, program documents and materials, and the implementers' final project reports also informed the case studies.

CHAPTER 3

Program Findings

This section describes findings from the 26 South Asia Region Development Marketplace (SARDM) implementers in designing and implementing interventions to address HIV stigma and discrimination. The research team's analytical approach involved both in-depth assessment, including case studies on six projects, and a broad look across the spectrum of implementer experience to distill lessons.

Findings across Programs

The most promising projects used various approaches to raise awareness about stigma and discrimination, such as correcting misinformation about HIV and marginalized populations, empowering marginalized groups, and addressing harmful norms and behaviors. No one formula can capture the diversity and ingenuity reflected in this body of work. But the findings do suggest some broad crosscutting principles, as well as programmatic and operational lessons associated with specific approaches.

In terms of broad lessons and principles, the experiences of all SARDM implementers suggest the following:

• *Community organizations achieved a great deal for relatively little investment.* The SARDM funding totaled US$1.04 million across 26 projects.

The results suggest that, combined, the projects reached more than 96,264 people; trained 4,905 people; led to 504 news articles; and developed 426 products such as training curricula, information, education and communication materials, documentaries, and plays. Community organizations, some of which had received no or little external support before, undertook new activities and developed new capacities despite the relatively small maximum grant size of US$40,000. Overall, the results suggest a high return on investment.

- *SARDM grants seeded considerable innovation.* Project approaches reflected enormous creativity, ranging from beauty pageants to restaurants run by sex workers. The grants led to new alliances, such as those between panchayat (local government) leaders and the Indian community organization Lotus Integrated AIDS Awareness Sangam. Grants also led to some unlikely partnerships, such as those between sex workers and the police. In Afghanistan, one project partnered with the government to support religious leaders in incorporating antistigma messaging into Friday prayers.

- *The most effective projects required substantial up-front planning and effort.* Regardless of the implementers' particular approach or the population served, the most promising projects invested considerable time and effort in engaging gatekeepers, conducting formative research on different audiences, training, forming new partnerships, and conducting other activities. Donors and practitioners interested in stigma reduction interventions should factor in sufficient up-front time and funding for such activities.

- *The most promising work used multiple strategies and stakeholders to address stigma.* Even where projects initially appeared to be single-focus interventions (for example, theater), successful implementation required a range of other activities, such as training, engagement with policy makers, and media relations.

- *Effective efforts were led by or continuously engaged marginalized communities.* Involving marginalized communities is essential for strengthening capacity, ensuring appropriate messaging, and maximizing results. Strategies that foster some interaction between marginalized communities and the public—either directly or through the mass media—can be powerful in inspiring change. Products such as films or plays that are developed by, or strongly reflect the input of, marginalized communities are likely to be more compelling to audiences and to enjoy rapid dissemination.

Lessons from Specific Program Approaches

This section describes lessons associated with specific programmatic approaches taken by implementers.

Engaging Gatekeepers and Opinion Leaders

In this report, *gatekeepers* are people or groups that control access to somebody or something. In project terms, gatekeepers permit entry into a given community or setting. *Opinion leaders* are influential members of a community group or society. Others turn to them for guidance, and their ideas and behavior serve as a model to others. Depending on the circumstances, someone could be both an opinion leader and a gatekeeper.

Encourage positive behavior change by inviting rather than indicting allies. Facing discriminatory laws and widespread abuse of their human rights, many marginalized populations perceive gatekeepers and opinion leaders as barriers rather than as potential allies. However, the most effective programs established direct connections with groups such as police, health care professionals, and religious leaders who had been avoided in the past. Project Baduku, an advocacy campaign led by three organizations of female sex workers in Bangalore, India, developed an effective strategy of engaging opinion leaders by approaching them with welcome—a "rose," in their words—rather than blame and condemnation. Their Rose campaign targeted police and health care professionals, groups that have particular influence over the treatment and well-being of sex workers. Their strategy was to reinforce positive behavior by presenting roses to police personnel and doctors who had demonstrated good behavior toward female sex workers. They also presented roses to people who had been particularly stigmatizing and abusive in the past to encourage behavior change among these individuals.

This simple and quick advocacy approach inspired cooperation and support and helped change negative attitudes and behaviors. Following the campaign, the number of stigma and discrimination cases female sex workers reported to the police grew from 0 to 11, all of which the police responded to and resolved. In addition, sex workers anecdotally reported less harassment and violence from the police following the intervention in a jurisdiction where violence had previously been high. Service use increased: the percentage of HIV-positive female sex workers regularly seeking care and treatment services at antiretroviral therapy (ART) centers in Bangalore increased from 30 percent before the project to 60 percent afterward. Also important, women appeared to be more comfortable sharing their HIV status with their families and project staff members. Overall, health care workers received the campaign positively. The head of the ART department at Victoria Hospital in Bangalore said that it was "motivating for the medical staff to see such dedication from the sex worker community. Since the campaign, we began advising women to go to the Lawyer's Collective to seek help for violence issues. We are also sending students for training at Swathi Mahila Sangha [one of the sex worker support organizations] to better understand the issues facing women in sex work."

Police can make unlikely, but powerful, partners. Ashodaya Samithi, an organization of HIV-positive and -negative sex workers in Mysore, India, engaged opinion leaders throughout its project. A key component of the intervention was establishing a restaurant owned and operated by sex workers to fight stigma and provide an additional source of income. To ensure the protection of the sex workers' rights, Ashodaya engaged the police from the inception of the project. Recognizing that police officers are often transferred to other locations, Ashodaya engaged in continuous advocacy, even becoming involved in cadet training. As a result, sex workers experienced reduced violence from the police during the project period. In addition, the police commissioner agreed to inaugurate the restaurant, representing a public statement of support for the sex worker community. This support led to more business for the restaurant, in terms of dine-in customers and catering requests from government offices throughout Mysore, and helped strengthen the sustainability of the restaurant and thus the care and support services provided to the community by Ashodaya. The restaurant typically serves more than 400 people a day.

Government partners can provide entrée to religious leaders and help spur broad engagement of faith-based communities in stigma reduction. Religious leaders play a critical role in shaping public opinion in much of the world, but relatively few organizations have effectively engaged them in addressing HIV stigma and discrimination. Taboo subjects, such as sexuality, often pose barriers to greater involvement of faith-based communities as advocates for HIV awareness and stigma reduction. With this in mind, four SARDM implementers—three in Afghanistan and one in India—used a strategy of working with the government at some level to gain access to religious leaders. For example, in Jalalabad, Afghanistan, the Afghan Help and Training Program (AHTP) developed a partnership with the government that spurred the involvement of *mullahs* and *mawlawies* (senior religious scholars) in a broad campaign to reduce stigma and discrimination. The Ministry of Haj and Religious Affairs and its provincial suboffices were involved in finalizing the seven-day training curriculum and selecting religious leaders to participate in the trainings. The National AIDS Control Program also reviewed and approved the training curriculum. Following approval from the government, the AHTP trained 10 mawlawies as master trainers. The master trainers then went on to train more than 300 mullahs and mawlawies on HIV and AIDS epidemiology and HIV-related stigma and discrimination.

Not only did this strategy cultivate a core of champions, but it also enabled broad and rapid diffusion of the stigma reduction messages. After the completion of the first round of training, religious leaders organized large gatherings of mullahs and mawlawies to raise awareness of HIV-related stigma and discrimination. These gatherings reached approximately 400 mullahs and mawlawies, who agreed to address HIV- and AIDS-related stigma and discrimination in their teachings. The AHTP then used print and broadcast media to further promote and reinforce the mullahs' messages about stigma and HIV and AIDS.

Using religious texts is an effective approach for strengthening commitment of religious leaders. Another strategy to cultivate champions among religious leaders involved using the Koran. One SARDM implementer, the Afghan Family Guidance Association (AFGA) in Kabul, used Koranic *suras* (verses) that call for compassion in trainings of religious leaders. In effect, this group contextualized the effort against stigma and discrimination in Koranic teachings. AFGA also provided specific guidance and reference materials for religious leaders, such as specific passages from the Koran that could be referenced to support antidiscrimination messages and incorporate lessons about HIV and stigma and discrimination into Friday prayer speeches (*khutba*). The project then went on to record and broadcast khutbas containing HIV stigma reduction messages on television.

Local political leaders are key to modeling nonstigmatizing behaviors.
Stigma and discrimination that occur in daily life are particularly damaging to marginalized groups. Local political leaders can be powerful change agents for addressing this issue. Local leaders in many communities, particularly rural ones, are often the first line of authority in local disputes, making them a potential key advocate for redress and justice. As with religious leaders, their communities look to them to set acceptable and appropriate social and behavioral norms. They hold power, both through their own actions and as justice channels, to reduce stigmatizing attitudes and discriminatory actions and to build acceptance for marginalized groups.

Recognizing this social structure, the Lotus project in southern India focused on village panchayat leaders as a means to catalyze stigma reduction. The project involved panchayat leaders throughout as respondents in baseline data collection, by obtaining their permission and support for the performance of the play in their village; as audience members; and finally, as a result of the play and interactions with Lotus members, as advocates for men who have sex with men (MSM) living in their villages. The project inspired changes in the behaviors and attitudes of panchayat leaders, which had a positive ripple effect on villagers under their authority. Reported changes included increased respect in daily interactions (from "he now greets me when he sees me" to "I am now treated with respect; he even invites me for tea and offers me a lift in his vehicle"). In a number of instances, panchayat leaders intervened to stop incidents of harassment or to ensure MSM or transgender village members could get access to government work schemes.

Buy-in from government is a precondition for successful project implementation and longer-term sustainability. By engaging with national and local government authorities early and continuously, many SARDM implementers have increased government interest in learning from their innovations, supporting replication and scale-up, and making stigma reduction a national priority. Some implementers worked effectively with different levels of government to further their goals. In India, Lotus had entrée to local panchayat leaders because it obtained a letter from the Tamil Nadu State AIDS Control Society. Many implementers involved national and local authorities in project start-up and inaugural events and throughout the course of the project (for example, in World AIDS Day activities). Some projects included officials in formal trainings—with powerful results. The Voluntary Health Association of Tripura implemented a range of project activities in the city of Agartala,

India, including stigma reduction training for panchayat members and Border Security Forces. As a result of the training, panchayat members took the initiative in organizing meetings to promote stigma reduction, and members of the Border Security Forces started referring people living with HIV to an ART center in Agartala. In fact, obtaining government buy-in was part of the SARDM approach in selecting implementers, because representatives from national AIDS programs were on the selection jury for the grants. As a result of this participation, the National AIDS Control Organisation (NACO) in India decided to sponsor, with the support of the United Nations Development Programme, 12 of the finalists from India that the SARDM was unable to support. Additionally, NACO is developing a national communications strategy to reduce stigma.

For an example of another successful project that required government cooperation, see box 3.1.

Box 3.1

Beauty and Brains

Men who have sex with men and transgender individuals are often stigmatized in Nepalese society, as in most societies. Part of this stigma is caused by a general lack of awareness and understanding about MSM and transgender individuals, as well as by the absence of clear language in the constitution to protect their rights. To address this gap, the Federation of Sexual and Gender Minorities Nepal (FSGMN), Blue Diamond Society, and other partners implemented an innovative advocacy campaign called "Beauty and Brains" throughout Nepal.

The intervention consisted of six beauty pageants, five regional and one national, to identify national and regional ambassadors among networks of MSM and transgender individuals. Pageant contestants received five days of preparatory training on public speaking, choreography, and interpersonal communication skills, as well as information regarding HIV and other sexually transmitted infections, human rights, and stigma and discrimination. Through songs, dance, drama, poems, and other performances in the competition, pageant contestants delivered messages about HIV prevention and other issues faced by the transgender community. Winners were selected on the basis of level of confidence, presentation, personality, and subject matter. The top three contestants from each region advanced to the national competition, where the national and regional ambassadors were selected.

(continued)

Box 3.1 *(continued)*

Five regional winners were declared and appointed as regional HIV ambassadors, and one contestant was declared the national ambassador. FSGMN then supported the ambassadors in leading a public advocacy campaign, a media campaign, and a political and constitutional rights campaign in their localities. These campaigns sought to promote the health and human rights of the transgender community by coordinating with local civil society organizations, human rights organizations, media, and organizations working on HIV and AIDS. Throughout the project, ambassadors participated in public forums, talk programs, seminars, and other gatherings to rally people around lesbian, gay, bisexual, transgender, and intersex issues and to support human rights.

The intervention had a number of positive outcomes. Foremost among them were the following:

- The establishment, on the national television station, of a weekly *Third Sex* program dedicated to promoting lesbian, gay, bisexual, transgender, and intersex human rights
- The inclusion of lesbian, gay, bisexual, transgender, and intersex human rights in political party manifestos and the promotion of these rights in the revised framework of the constitution
- The Nepalese government's first-time allocation of more than NrP 3 million in the fiscal year 2009/10 budget for the promotion of lesbian, gay, bisexual, transgender, and intersex human rights
- A partnership with Save the Children; the Family Planning Association of Nepal; and the Global Fund to Fight AIDS, Tuberculosis, and Malaria to implement HIV prevention programs for MSM and transgender individuals in 14 districts in Nepal. This partnership currently employs four of the regional ambassadors and 200 members of the MSM and transgender communities.

The success of this intervention was in large part because of the strong relationships that FSGMN built with key stakeholders, including government officials, at the beginning of the project and FSGMN's consistent engagement with these stakeholders throughout project implementation.

Source: Federation of Sexual and Gender Minorities Nepal.

Strengthening the Capacity of Marginalized Populations to Address Stigma

Finding ways to strengthen the capacity of marginalized populations to address stigma was an important component of many of the programs.

Improving self-efficacy and reducing self-stigma among marginalized populations are key to strengthening capacity. To effectively involve marginalized populations in stigma reduction efforts, a number of projects incorporated approaches to address the pernicious effects of *self-stigma*, or the internalization of society's negative attitudes. Self-stigma is linked to both depression and self-destructive behavior. In terms of program efforts, it can reduce uptake of protective behavior, deter care seeking, and result in poor adherence to medication regimens. Because self-stigma is also connected to social isolation, it can deter engagement in support networks and activities addressing HIV stigma and discrimination. Project experience suggests that the interaction of people living with HIV and the public can be a powerful force for change, though people need to be willing to engage publicly for this strategy to work.

Addressing self-stigma effectively is an important precondition for effective engagement of marginalized communities and for project success. Building and practicing new skills are efficient ways to strengthen self-efficacy, reduce self-stigma, and heighten engagement in HIV efforts. For example, a performer in the theater troupe supported by the Indian organization We Care Social Service Society expressed how participating in the plays empowered him to support others:

> When I am providing the information [in the play], it makes me feel stronger as I am telling people they can live long with HIV if they take medicine, and so that reinforces that for me and encourages me to do that. When I disclose my status on stage, afterwards it leads to [people living with HIV] coming to talk to me, and I can help them with information and referral to services like We Care, and it makes me feel good to be able to help them. Nearly 15 people have disclosed [their status] to me after the plays. I also feel good to share that I got infected through sharing needles and that when I was doing this I did not know it could bring HIV. By sharing this information, hopefully I can prevent others getting infected this way.

Similarly, a woman living with HIV trained in interviewing as part of The Communication Hub's project activities explained how she gained confidence through the process:

> I have always been the interviewee, not the person doing the interviews. . . . Now I understand all these technical things—for example, differences between conducting interviews in the field and in the studio. I feel really good about being in the position to ask the questions, since I am always answering questions. But I also learned a lot about how difficult it is to do good interviews, that there are lots of skills needed.

Connections with support communities are critical. A number of implementer activities provided immediate access to support networks for
members of marginalized populations who previously thought they were
alone. Evidence gathered from community-led interventions highlights
the critical role that supportive networks play in helping strengthen
capacity of marginalized communities to reduce stigma and discrimination. In a community where a play focusing on stigma reduction toward
MSM was performed, one man explained:

> Before, when I was teased in my village, I was afraid to talk back because I was
> alone and I was afraid [people] would come and attack me. After the play, some
> boys gathered around me to tell me a play had occurred and it was about MSM,
> and the boys said they now understood and apologized for what they had done.
> Now I felt I could speak back and also told the boys that now you see I belong
> to a big group and so if something happens to me, I have a group to support
> me and my rights. Now there is no more teasing in my village from the youth.

*Strategic partnerships are important for greater learning and effective-
ness.* Many projects worked closely with local networks of people living
with HIV or other groups experiencing stigma to ensure program strategies and messages were appropriate at addressing the needs and concerns
of the target population. The Communication Hub, a development communication firm in Mumbai, partnered with the Network of Maharashtra
People Living with HIV from the inception of their project to harness
radio to empower people living with HIV and transform attitudes. Both
parties felt the partnership was central to the success of the project and
emphasized its importance in terms of the benefits, learning, and inspiration it brought to each of them. Both The Communication Hub and the
Network of Maharashtra People Living with HIV emphasized that key to
this successful partnership was communication, joint decision making,
and respect for the opinions of everyone involved.

Economically Empowering Marginalized Communities to Reduce Stigma and Discrimination

To reduce stigma and discrimination, marginalized communities must be
able to overcome economic challenges.

*Generating economic opportunities can reduce stigma on multiple
fronts.* Vulnerable populations often face economic challenges, such
as difficulty securing employment, that increase their exposure to

HIV risk. Poverty or lack of economic opportunity may heighten their likelihood of engaging in high-risk behaviors such as unprotected transactional sex and can reduce their ability to negotiate condom use with partners. A number of SARDM implementers addressed economic hardship by incorporating innovative economic empowerment elements to enhance stigma reduction and HIV prevention. Some groups offered economic empowerment programs, while others hired vulnerable people to implement program activities. Nine implementers, including Alliance Lanka, Ashodaya Samithi, Job Opportunity and Business Support (JOBS), Lanka+, Lotus, Saral, Swathi Mahila Sangha (SMS),[1] The Communication Hub, and We Care, provided vulnerable populations with opportunities to strengthen their economic stability.

By building skills and capacity and providing employment opportunities, several SARDM projects helped combat the perception that vulnerable populations cannot contribute to their families and society. Shifting this perception led to reduced stigma within both their families and their communities. A panchayat leader who saw a play about MSM explained:

> The play showed that [MSM] . . . have very special talents and that they can live with a profession and that they don't have to just live by alms. They can be self-sufficient, if they can live with self-esteem and contribute to society. I think that men who have sex with men should be treated equally and they should be given more skills and trade so they can live independently and live with self-esteem.

A block-batik trainer involved in the JOBS project in Bangladesh highlighted how the training empowered the former drug users who participated: "[The men] were very motivated and had a sense of pride at being able to create something. [The block-batik training] empowered them. . . . It was important for me to respect their opinions."

Another benefit of projects that include an income-generating opportunity is that they often enhance long-term sustainability. For example, Ashodaya Samithi reinvested project-generated income to expand services to network members and to enhance stigma reduction and advocacy efforts. In addition, income earned by individuals, such as former drug users who participated in the JOBS project, afforded the men an opportunity to contribute to their families and save money, both of which strengthened confidence and inspired the men to stay drug free.

Economic empowerment approaches can inspire greater engagement among vulnerable populations in stigma reduction and HIV prevention. After taking advantage of economic opportunities made possible through the interventions, a number of beneficiaries became stigma reduction advocates in their communities, further diffusing the project messages and encouraging others to take protective behaviors. For example, a former drug user who participated in the JOBS project highlighted how he shared the information he learned about HIV with other drug users in his community:

> Since I joined the JOBS project, I have been away from drugs. I also learned a lot about HIV and gained some technical skills. I am now very careful in my sex life. I inform other drug users about HIV and how to protect themselves. . . . I tell them to spend the three taka to buy clean needles instead of sharing. I also tell them about using condoms during sex.

This type of peer education, which was documented across the projects that used economic empowerment approaches, was an unintended positive outcome of these interventions.

Using Cultural Art Forms to Reduce Stigma
Theater, music, dance, and other cultural art forms proved to be an effective way to bring messages about HIV prevention, care, and treatment and the stigma and discrimination faced by vulnerable populations to the general community.

Cultural approaches can foster empathy in audiences, which is key in reducing stigmatizing attitudes and behaviors. Important drivers of HIV stigma include fears of casual transmission and culturally rooted attitudes about gender, sexuality, sex work, drug use, and other characteristics. An important way of addressing these fears and attitudes involves promoting empathy in audiences or helping people understand how they share many values and goals with marginalized groups, including the desire to be accepted and to contribute to family and society. This understanding or identification, in turn, appears to be key in inspiring more positive attitudes and behaviors toward marginalized populations.

Several SARDM projects used the strategy of creating empathy through traditional art forms. Using theater, music, and dance, the projects engaged community members in discussions about HIV transmission and prevention, stigma and discrimination, and the particular challenges faced by people living with HIV and other marginalized groups. These approaches often offered opportunities for the public to interact with marginalized people, which enhanced empathy and identification. A number of projects purposely designed opportunities for discussion into their performances.

In Kancheepuram district, India, We Care Social Service Society, a community-based nongovernmental organization (NGO), promoted community discussion and debate about HIV stigma and discrimination using a traditional folk media known as *therukoothu* (street drama). The play, divided into three segments of one hour each, included messages about living with HIV, the harmful effects of stigma and discrimination, and HIV transmission and prevention. At several points, the play stopped to allow the audience to ask questions and to allow actors to ask the audience questions; prizes were awarded to those who actively participated. The theater troupe resided in the village during the performance period (a total of four days), which provided additional opportunities for interaction with villagers. A key lesson from this intervention was the power of theater to raise sensitive issues with a diverse audience. Many villagers expressed gratitude for having received new information on HIV. They spoke of the fears they had prior to the play about contracting HIV through casual means and how such fear led to discrimination against people living with HIV. One young man explained that "definitely behavior toward people living with HIV will change because we no longer are afraid of them. My own behavior will definitely change as I am no longer afraid."

Cultural approaches rooted in life experience tend to be more powerful.
An important factor in Lotus's success was that the play Lotus offered was developed and performed by MSM. The plot line derived directly from the life experience of the author. The story, focused on a family's efforts to force the son into marriage, dramatizes a high-tension and familiar scenario for MSM. Lotus also conducted considerable research with MSM about their experiences of stigma and with its key target audience, panchayat leaders. Lotus then incorporated what it learned into the storyline. This research helped Lotus write a story for maximum effect on these leaders and others, who recognized their role in perpetuating stigmatizing attitudes and behaviors. This reflection of people's real-life experiences, combined with enormous care and effort in crafting the script, helped make the play entertaining, informative, and persuasive. The performances drew large, multigenerational crowds.

Box 3.2

Using Theater to Teach Tolerance

Men who have sex with men often face intense challenges at home. As the director of Lotus Integrated AIDS Awareness Sangam, a Tamil Nadu–based organization, tells it, "If it became known that someone was a sexual minority and he was kicked out of the house by his parents, he would have to get involved in sex work and begging."

Lotus developed a play to dramatize these challenges and to provide a more positive ending than real life often delivers. In the story, a son faces intense pressure from his parents to get married. When he expresses reluctance, his father responds, "Only if a girl comes to a house, lights a lamp,[a] and gives birth to grandchildren can we stand with our head held high in our community."

One of the most powerful parts of the play is when the son, facing rejection from family, friends, and community members, expresses his despondency. The audience tends to go completely silent when he says, "They tease me by calling me *ombathu*[b] . . . God! Why did you give me a life like this?"

This part of the play, as well as the many instances of hurtful treatment the story depicts, resonates strongly with audience members. After performances, cast members and others recount being approached by community members, who apologize to them for past mistreatment.

The play also helped audience members understand how they could be more supportive toward men with a different sexual orientation. In one scene, a potential bride for the son explains to the son's parents, "I have studied psychology and nursing. And there's no doubt about it. He's a man with the thoughts and feelings of a woman. Please don't waste his life by getting him married or waste the life of another woman in so doing."

Later, a counselor reinforces with the parents the need for acceptance and respect. He tells them, "Like any man or woman, an effeminate man is born naturally. If he is given due respect and recognition in family and society, he can also achieve many things in his life."

In the end, the father speaks to his son with new understanding, telling him he should choose the life he wishes to have.

Source: Lotus Integrated AIDS Awareness Sangam.
a. In Tamil Nadu, a tradition exists in which a newlywed bride enters the home of her husband and lights a lamp.
b. "Number 9"—a popular derogatory slang word for effeminate men.

Real-life experiences also strengthened the power of a music and dance series developed in West Bengal, India, by the local organization Society for Positive Atmosphere and Related Support to HIV/AIDS. The series consisted of three weekly performances by Baul singers, traditional singing troupes that provide entertainment in West Bengal. The first performance focused on how HIV is transmitted, the second on personal experiences of people living with HIV in the community, and the third on the importance of care and support for people living with HIV. Some participants considered the second session the most engaging. To develop the second performance, the Baul singers, mostly local farmers, collaborated with a community health worker living with HIV to create a song about her experiences with HIV and discrimination. Before and after each performance, the community health worker and the district team leader (who did not have HIV) led a group discussion with community members attending the performance that allowed them to ask questions and interact with a person living with HIV. This mode of message delivery powerfully affected community members and was also well received by community members living with HIV and their families. The HIV songs were so popular that Baul singers reported receiving requests to perform them at village events well after the intervention had ended.

Cultural approaches can appeal to positive values to inspire behavior change. We Care found that the power of its play was knowing the audience and crafting messages that responded specifically to villagers' knowledge gaps about HIV, as well as appealing to villagers' fundamental desire to help family and community members. In these villages, fear of casual transmission of HIV was prevalent before the play. Because few villagers knew about ART, few realized that people living with HIV can have a productive, healthy life. The play not only addressed information gaps but also appealed to the villagers' sense of compassion and desire to support family and community members. After the play, villagers talked about how they had not realized what stigma and discrimination did and how they now understood and would no longer practice stigma and discrimination. They also talked at length about the importance of supporting people living with HIV so that they could lead healthy and productive lives.

Cultural approaches are effective in broaching taboo subjects. Overall, implementers using cultural approaches found they were able to more readily broach issues such as sexuality and drug use, thereby opening up public discussion and inspiring reconsideration of broadly held myths and misconceptions. Lotus, for example, crafted its play to address the highly sensitive issue of MSM and transgender persons in a way that would not offend or threaten, but rather draw in the audience to understand the issues and the negative effects of stigma and discrimination. In addition, the preparation time spent ahead of the performance in each village and formal and informal opportunities created at the end of the intervention to ask questions and interact one on one with the performers allowed discussion and exchange on issues the performance raised, thus providing a nonthreatening and socially acceptable way to broach sensitive and taboo topics. Spectators were able to interact directly with the performers—nearly all MSM—thereby dispelling myths and promoting comprehension of the play's key messages. Typically, audience members had never interacted with anyone living with HIV or in a respectful way with MSM. For the performers, the experience of being directly involved in advocacy and seeing immediate, positive reactions from community members was empowering.

Harnessing Mass Media to Reduce Stigma

Traditional media, such as radio, television, and the press, can be powerful tools in efforts to reduce stigma.

Media approaches offer multiple avenues for reducing stigma but also some serious potential pitfalls. Several projects engaged the media effectively in their stigma reduction efforts. This involvement took one of three forms. Some groups, including Afghan Family Guidance Association, Nari Unnayan Shakti, Pakistan Press Foundation, and Voluntary Health Association of Tripura, trained journalists about stigma and discrimination and ways to report in nonstigmatizing ways. Other groups, including Afghan Family Guidance Association, Federation of Sexual and Gender Minorities Nepal, Lotus, and Swathi Mahila Sanga, engaged with the media at key points in project implementation to amplify the reach of their efforts. Last, Sai Paranjpye and a few groups, such as Concern Worldwide, Drik Picture Library, and The Communication Hub, developed media products such as training films, documentaries, and radio documentaries to be used as stigma reduction tools.

Given the sensitive subject matter and vulnerability of marginalized groups, media approaches present some challenges. Anyone who participates in awareness-raising activities with journalists needs to understand the possible ramifications of sharing his or her story publicly. Working with children to share their stories requires extra care to ensure that participation is voluntary on the part of the child and that the child and parents or guardians fully understand the potential ramifications of involvement. Support systems should be in place to help participants cope with public disclosure. Spokespeople for media activities need to be thoroughly prepared for difficult questions. In general, projects need to devote considerable time to engage and sensitize journalists. Few reporters could write about stigma and discrimination in an effective, nonsensational way without training. In some cases, largely because of high levels of stigma, projects had difficulty finding people willing to share their stories publicly through the media. Participation can be encouraged, however, through strong connections to networks and support groups.

People living with HIV can inspire journalists to eliminate stigmatizing language and stories. The language and images portrayed in print and broadcast media often unintentionally foster stigma and discrimination toward people living with HIV and groups considered particularly vulnerable to HIV infection. In an effort to ensure that journalists were fighting stigma instead of propagating it, four SARDM implementers adapted existing training curricula to sensitize members of the media about HIV, AIDS, and stigma and discrimination. The active participation of people living with HIV can make these efforts especially powerful. The organization Nari Unnayan Shakti conducted a two-day training for more than 130 journalists in six cities throughout Bangladesh. According to the project directors, the involvement of people living with HIV in raising awareness about stigma and discrimination was critical. The prevalence of HIV is quite low in Bangladesh, and many of the journalists had never engaged with a person living with HIV before, so the opportunity to do so helped them overcome their own fears and misconceptions and also helped them understand the stigma and discrimination that people with HIV face. The project helped journalists channel their new understanding into actual articles. By the end of the project period, 78 (57 percent) of the journalists trained had published articles in their local papers.

Partnering with media-savvy groups can optimize results of media efforts. Good press coverage can enhance the reach and influence of public health messages, but often community-led organizations do not have enough media relations experience to maximize this potential. Securing strong coverage of key project messages, especially on sensitive and easily sensationalized subjects, likely requires the help of partners with media relations expertise. To this end, Swathi Mahila Sangha solicited the Centre for Advocacy and Research (CFAR) to prepare female sex workers living with HIV for various media events that were part of an advocacy campaign in India. The support received from CFAR led to one sex worker participating in a television interview, two giving radio interviews, and six participating together in a live press conference to reduce stigma and discrimination among the public and journalists. For the press conference, the women had only three minutes each to get their message across, so messages had to be carefully crafted and practiced. They were also coached on how to respond to questions that might be direct and even offensive or stigmatizing. The staff person who helped train and prepare the women for these media events noted how far the three sex worker organizations had come during the yearlong project period, from no engagement with the media to about 40 percent engagement. He also noted that "to have discourse with the media, you need to have a partnership with the media. Once you have discourse, the press can be used as a tool to promote your messages."

The media events that the team organized resulted in positive reactions from both journalists and the public. One of the community mobilizers living with HIV who participated in a television interview expressed how the advocacy project helped her become an advocate for others:

> I used to be ashamed and hide my [HIV] status. The project has helped me to overcome my own stigma. It has given me courage, and I am now comfortable sharing my status publicly. By boldly facing society, I can be a role model for other sex workers and help to stand up for their rights. Women should keep their heads high; that spirit brings me here every day [to work for the project].

Training for civil society organizations on media relations is often essential. Another key gap addressed by one of the SARDM implementers is the lack of capacity among many NGOs to properly engage with the media. These skills are critical to build the media relationships necessary for expanding reach of key messages and program outcomes. The Pakistan Press Foundation sought to strengthen the capacity of civil society professionals in Pakistan to work effectively with the media in reducing HIV-related stigma and discrimination. To accomplish this goal, the foundation organized five three-day training workshops, "Working with the Media," for civil society organizations in the cities of Abbottabad, Karachi, Lahore, and Quetta. Participation reached 119 civil society professionals from a range of civil society organizations, including NGOs working with the groups most at risk, adolescents, and those involved in general HIV awareness–raising activities. The purpose of the workshops was to train NGOs how to liaise with the media about their activities through press releases and letters to the editor. A key component of the workshop was a panel discussion in which civil society professionals engaged directly with experienced print and electronic journalists. By the end of the project, training participants had produced 187 press releases and letters to the editor.

Films, documentaries, and other products can ensure consistent quality and continuous diffusion of messages. Different forms of media can be used as stigma reduction tools. Packaging films, documentaries, and other products for widespread use allows quality control of messaging and continuous diffusion as other groups use the products after the project ends. Several of the SARDM implementers developed media to promote awareness about stigma and discrimination, share stories of experiences of stigma faced by people living with HIV, and address the specific challenges that marginalized groups faced. Concern Worldwide, in partnership with ActionAid Afghanistan and Just Afghan Capacity and Knowledge, produced six films on stigma and HIV and AIDS in two local Afghan languages (Pashto and Dari). The films were based on formative research among individuals living with HIV and AIDS in Kabul. Target groups for dissemination of the documentaries and training films included mullahs, teachers, prison and police officers, community leaders, and health professionals across districts and urban centers in Afghanistan. These films are now available for use by appropriate organizations and the National AIDS Control Program.

To address the specific HIV- and stigma-related issues facing truck drivers and injecting drug users in India, Sai Paranjpye produced two short films. The scripts for these films were produced in close consultation with members of the marginalized groups they were portraying. The films are enjoying extensive dissemination, through both the efforts of the filmmaker and wide use by other organizations. One of the films, *Suee* (*The Needle*), debuted in Mumbai in July 2009 and was hosted by the Narcotics Control Bureau. The film also was shown at the International Conference on AIDS in Asia and the Pacific in Bali, Indonesia, in July 2009 and at the International Harm Reduction Conference film festival in Liverpool, United Kingdom, in May 2010. Organizations that have acquired the film for screening include Air Headquarters, Anand Foundation, Johnson & Johnson, Muktangan, the Narcotics Control Bureau, Sangram Sangli, Sankalp Drug Rehabilitation Foundation, the Sharan and Humana People to People Foundation, and Tata Motors.

The other film, *Horrn Pukare* (*Call of the Horn*), is being shown throughout truck drivers' networks through the Transport Corporation of India. Screenings are followed by workshops and interactive sessions with facilitators. A local organization in Nigdi shows the film regularly as part of its HIV and AIDS awareness drives. The ICICI Bank and the Mehandale Transport Group of Pune also show the film during workshops. An English-subtitled DVD (digital video disc) version of the film has been sent to the AIDS Prevention and Control Project in Tamil Nadu, the Mumbai District AIDS Control Society, and the National AIDS Control Organisation of India. The World Bank lends both films to development partners for internal viewing and training purposes.

Mass media can raise the profile of an issue through broad reach and active word of mouth. ISTV Network and the Institute of Social Work and Research produced a televised game show that enjoyed a broad audience and generated positive word of mouth. In the game show, which aired in Manipur, India, a host posed HIV-related questions to contestants in a "hot seat." People were rewarded for answering correctly. The questions, developed by experts and practitioners, were designed to reduce fears and misconceptions related to HIV and to reduce stigma. People living with HIV or others who have experienced stigma also participated in answering questions. Working with the Manipur Network of People Living with HIV, the project developed special episodes featuring only people living with HIV. The host, by hugging and shaking hands with contestants, reinforced the message that HIV is not transmitted through casual contact. A total of 68 episodes aired across four districts to an estimated half million viewers. The end-line survey suggests the show also fostered word of mouth, with about 7 in 10 viewers reporting they discussed the program with friends and family members. Word of mouth can be especially powerful because information conveyed through family and friends is often more deeply processed and more likely to be accepted and internalized. The end-line survey also indicates that the vast majority of viewers thought the game show educated viewers and reduced HIV stigma and discrimination.

Participating in media initiatives can be empowering for marginalized populations. A chief executive of The Communication Hub described their goal:

> We are surrounded by the negative . . . newspapers, TV, radio . . . and most of HIV/AIDS news again brings depressing, albeit real, stories to us. But for every one person who stigmatizes, there is someone who cares! We wanted to talk about them, share their stories, listen to them, get inspired by them, celebrate them.

This rationale was the inspiration for The Communication Hub's project, which trained people living with HIV to conduct joint interviews in their communities with the HIV-positive person and the HIV-negative support person identified as key in that person's life. The interviews captured personal stories about compassion, care, and support for people living with HIV from their families and communities. The idea was to showcase role models who do not stigmatize and share their experiences and stories throughout rural and semi-rural areas through radio. The interview experience turned out to be an empowering one for all involved. One young man living with HIV, who was interviewed together with a close friend who is HIV negative, explained his experience of participating this way:

> To be frank, when I first came to know [about the possibility of doing an interview] I was scared, but then I thought about it and thought if by telling my story I can reach all people in Maharashtra, this will help reduce stigma, and so I should do it. And those who are negative will begin to think that they need to help people living with HIV . . . and this will help reduce stigma. I got the very great opportunity, I can reach many people with my story and reduce stigma, [and] it makes me feel good.

Note

1. Implementing partners included Swathi Mahila Sangha, Vijaya Mahila Sangha, Jyothi Mahila Sangha, and the Swasti Health Resource Center. Because the SARDM funding was channeled through SMS and for ease of reading, only SMS is listed as the implementing organization here and elsewhere in this report.

CHAPTER 4

Capacity-Strengthening Efforts and Lessons Learned

The South Asia Region Development Marketplace (SARDM) implementers reflected a range of organizations, including small, community-based organizations, larger international nongovernmental organizations (NGOs), networks of men who have sex with men, and transgender and sex worker communities. They also had varying levels of experience in designing projects, implementing interventions, and assessing their effectiveness. With support from SARDM, the International Center for Research on Women (ICRW) provided assistance to the implementers to strengthen their capacity in a range of areas and through different mechanisms.

Types of Capacity-Strengthening Support and Technical Assistance Provided to Implementers

Formal group training and assistance occurred at three points during the 18-month period, beginning with two half-day sessions for implementers during the initial Development Marketplace event, held in May 2008, to select the finalists. These sessions reviewed current stigma reduction principles based on existing information from pilot programs around the globe, basic principles of monitoring and evaluation, and specific guidance on available indicators (see box 4.1) for assessing stigma reduction interventions (Tanzania Stigma-Indicators Field Testing Group 2005).

The ICRW research team provided SARDM implementers with tools for stigma reduction and monitoring and evaluation (M&E) as well as references to other available stigma reduction tools. In addition, each group received individual attention to review its proposed activities for feasibility

---

Box 4.1

Indicators That Can Be Used to Assess Stigma at the Community Level

Fear

Fear of HIV transmission through day-to-day contact can be assessed by asking whether individuals fear contracting HIV in the following situations:

- If they touch the saliva of a person living with HIV or AIDS
- If they touch the sweat of a person living with HIV or AIDS
- If they touch the excreta of a person living with HIV or AIDS
- If they eat food prepared by a person living with HIV or AIDS.

In addition, fear of HIV transmission to a child can be assessed by asking whether individuals fear their child would become infected with HIV from playing with a child who has HIV or AIDS.

Shame and Blame

Stigma and discrimination based on shame, blame, and judgment can be determined by assessing agreement with the following statements:

Shame

- I would feel ashamed if I were infected with HIV.
- People with HIV or AIDS should be ashamed of themselves.
- I would be ashamed if someone in my family had HIV or AIDS.

Blame and judgment

- It is women prostitutes who spread HIV in our community.
- HIV is a punishment for bad behavior.
- People living with HIV or AIDS are promiscuous.
- HIV is a punishment from God.

(continued)

Box 4.1 *(continued)*

Discrimination (Enacted Stigma)

The level of discrimination can be assessed by asking people whether they are aware of or have seen incidents during which a person living with HIV or AIDS experienced the following:

Isolation (including physical and social exclusion)

- Being excluded from a social gathering
- Being abandoned by a partner
- Being abandoned or sent away by family members.

Verbal stigma

- Being teased, insulted, or sworn at
- Being gossiped about.

Loss of identity or role

- Losing respect or standing within the family, the community, or both

Loss of access to resources or services

- Losing customers or a job
- Having property taken away
- Being denied health care services, social services, or education.

Source: UNAIDS 2007.

and alignment with best practices. In September 2008, additional training was provided on stigma messaging and terminology to implementers whose projects included a media or communications component. In December 2008, the ICRW led a four-day M&E workshop in New Delhi, where the implementers learned how to prepare logic models and M&E plans in direct consultation with technical experts and other SARDM implementers. The workshop also provided an opportunity to reflect on implementation progress to date and discuss challenges and potential solutions with fellow implementers and the larger SARDM team. The workshop reinforced stigma reduction practices by sharing a key stigma reduction programming tool, *Understanding and Challenging HIV Stigma: Toolkit for Action* (AED, ICRW, and International HIV/AIDS Alliance 2007).

In addition to the structured group trainings, when requested the ICRW provided direct technical assistance to implementers for both their intervention and their M&E components. For example, the ICRW reviewed film scripts, billboard content, game show questions, training materials, baseline surveys, and pre- and posttraining evaluations. In addition, following the regional workshop, the ICRW helped individual SARDM implementers finalize their M&E plans.

Recommendations for Strengthening Programmatic and M&E Capacity

Several lessons learned through the process of strengthening capacity and providing technical assistance to these large and diverse groups of program implementers can be used to inform other grants programs working on stigma or similarly nascent areas of work:

- *Capacity strengthening should be a continuous process for long-term sustainability.* As a result of SARDM support, most implementers gained a basic knowledge of M&E principles and increased their capacity to collect formative and monitoring data to strengthen program implementation, record outcomes, and document key process issues to facilitate sharing lessons learned. A logical next step in capacity strengthening for a number of implementers, particularly if their programs are scaled up, would be more intensive technical support to undertake quantitative impact evaluation of their programs, which would provide the type of evidence many large donors seek before making a sizable investment.
- *M&E training and support should be tailored to implementers' capacity and experience.* The SARDM implementers varied widely in terms of experience and capacity to conduct program M&E. Although some implementers were larger, international NGOs, others had never received external funding before. This variation in experience greatly enriched collective learning. It also gives rise to some suggestions for future initiatives aiming to support and document innovations to reduce stigma and discrimination. First, early and up-front training and technical assistance on the basics of M&E are important. The approach should be comprehensive, catering to the wide variation in experience of community groups and networks. For example, a three- to five-day training could cover all relevant information, including best practices for program and intervention design as well as M&E

basics, and provide ample time for implementers to work with technical experts to develop program logic models and M&E plans. Second, in addition to up-front training, a mix of proactive and on-demand technical assistance could be effective. Experienced groups are more likely to seek support actively, whereas others groups may need more assistance to identify and define their needs. Finally, technical assistance to implementers could support alignment of M&E and data collection with funding levels, capacity, and time frame.

- *Programmatic technical assistance is critical.* In working with nascent topic areas such as stigma reduction, in addition to capacity strengthening in M&E, support (such as basic training and skills-building sessions) in programming and accessing existing best practices, programmatic tools, and intervention models will strengthen implementers' ability to achieve results. In HIV and AIDS work, messaging is a particular area in which a review of fundamental principles is critical. Despite best intentions, programs may unintentionally reinforce stigma and discrimination through language and images. Although this issue is of particular importance to media-related projects, all program materials (training, leaflets, and the like) should be reviewed to ensure that no inadvertent harm is being done through language and images.

References

AED (Academy for Educational Development), ICRW (International Center for Research on Women), and International HIV/AIDS Alliance. 2007. *Understanding and Challenging HIV Stigma: Toolkit for Action.* Rev. ed. Hove, U.K.: International HIV/AIDS Alliance. http://www.icrw.org/html/projects/stigma.html.

Tanzania Stigma-Indicators Field Testing Group. 2005. *Measuring HIV Stigma: Results of a Field Test in Tanzania.* Working report produced for review by the United States Agency for International Development. Washington, DC: International Center for Research on Women. http://www.icrw.org/publications/Working-Report-Measuring-HIV-Stigma-Results-of-Field-Test-in-Tanzania.pdf

UNAIDS (Joint United Nations Programme on HIV/AIDS). 2007. *Reducing HIV Stigma and Discrimination: A Critical Part of National AIDS Programmes—A Resource for National Stakeholders in the HIV Response.* Geneva: UNAIDS. http://data.unaids.org/pub/Report/2008/JC1521_stigmatisation_en.pdf.

CHAPTER 5

Recommendations for Action

The South Asia Region Development Marketplace (SARDM) implementers addressed different dimensions of HIV stigma and discrimination from a range of entry points. This body of experience provides a strong foundation for further stigma reduction efforts in the region and globally. Important next steps include actions to intensify and expand the response to stigma and discrimination. The following recommendations outline action steps for governments, donors, and practitioners.

Promote Intensified Government Support for a Scaled-Up Response to Stigma and Discrimination

Government support proved essential for SARDM implementers, giving them credibility, entrée to influential individuals, and ability to implement projects on sensitive issues. For smaller-scale efforts, government support, at least at the central level, does not necessarily need to be intensive. Even a relatively small item such as a letter of support can make a large difference to community organizations in implementing local interventions.

When the scale of activities increases, however, more intensified government involvement is key. The Afghan Family Guidance Association's close collaboration with the government, for example, greatly increased the reach of the association's stigma reduction efforts with religious leaders. This group worked with ministries in public health and religious affairs, including the National AIDS Control Program, to develop training and communications material. The government selected three senior religious leaders, who advise the Ministry of Haj and Religious Affairs, to work with the project to initiate a cascading training-of-trainers (TOT) program, resulting in the training of more than 100 mullahs. The General Directorate of Mosques of the Ministry of Haj and Religious Affairs formally disseminated key project messages about HIV stigma and discrimination to mosques for use in Friday prayers. Television channels, including the national channel, then broadcast these messages to an even larger public.

Promote Government Adoption of Stigma Reduction Efforts in Health Care

Stigma within health care settings can be especially severe for marginalized populations. They may be refused services, denied medicine, passed from provider to provider, and tested for HIV or have their serostatus disclosed without consent. Fortunately, tested approaches and tools exist for reducing discrimination in health care settings. A number of SARDM implementers also addressed these issues by adapting training materials and piloting intervention models that governments could consider for further refinement and possible adoption. Ashodaya Samithi, for example, collaborated with hospitals to improve quality of care for sex workers. The initiative involved training both health care providers and sex worker volunteers to help other sex workers access and navigate hospital care. Initial results have been promising: sex workers found hospital staff members more sensitive and attentive to their needs when accompanied by the volunteers. Use of health services by sex workers also increased. Another implementer, the National NGOs Network Group against AIDS–Nepal (Nangan), worked with hospitals, using a TOT approach to train all staff members on stigma reduction.

Encourage Replication of Promising Approaches through Organization-to-Organization Knowledge Transfer

In the process of implementation, SARDM implementers developed or deepened expertise in areas such as street theater, media relations, and stigma reduction training. Groups such as Lotus Integrated AIDS Awareness Sangam, Nari Unnayan Shakti, the New Light AIDS Control

Society, the Pakistan Press Foundation, Swathi Mahila Sangha, and The Communication Hub could help train other community organizations, including growing networks of marginalized populations, in conducting similar interventions. As part of this process, they could document their approach and strategies, thereby creating guidance and tools for others to replicate these activities. Guidance on approaches that offer more potential for scale and influence may be particularly useful. The New Light AIDS Control Society in Pakistan, for example, implemented a TOT effort that trained nearly 400 people, including men who have sex with men (MSM), health providers, and journalists.

Promote Use of Multipronged Programming Strategies for Increased Effectiveness

The most effective projects tended to offer services and activities that met multiple needs of marginalized populations. Ashodaya Samithi, for instance, addressed institutional stigma in Indian health care settings and offered sex workers access to support services and economic opportunities. Another example is Lotus Sangam, which implemented street theater performances in India to reduce stigmatizing attitudes among community members. These performances also let hard-to-reach MSM know they could access more information and services from Lotus, including counseling and group support. A broad HIV awareness and stigma reduction campaign that New Light AIDS Control Society developed, coupled with strengthening of referral systems and links for treatment and care services for MSM and transgender individuals, resulted in more than 350 new counseling clients. Reliance on a single approach such as employment training, without corresponding stigma reduction efforts or links to services, will be less effective.

Leverage Cultural and Media Efforts of SARDM Implementers to Maximize Reach and Results

Cultural and media products developed by SARDM implementers can be used by other groups to further spread stigma and discrimination reduction messages in different regions or populations in a given country.

Package Live Cultural Activities into Scalable Products

SARDM implementers such as Lotus, We Care Social Service Society, and the Society for Positive Atmosphere and Related Support to HIV/AIDS

(SPARSHA) invested considerable time and effort in developing compelling plays and performances. Packaging these efforts into products such as films or videos could diffuse messages even more widely. At least in one case, such extension is already taking place among SARDM implementers. The "Beauty and the Brain" pageant, led by the Federation of Sexual and Gender Minorities Nepal, is already the subject of a documentary.

Support Further Dissemination and Impact Evaluation of Media Products

The Communication Hub in Maharashtra, India, developed a promising 13-part radio series but initially lacked the budget to secure broadcast airtime and evaluate its effect. However, the Maharashtra State AIDS Control Society has recently included the program in its next financial year media budget (April 2010–March 2011). Hence, the project team anticipates the serial will be broadcast over the coming year. Including an evaluation component in the rollout would provide much-needed evidence on the effectiveness of such radio serials in shifting the underlying fears and attitudes that drive stigma and discrimination. The films on stigma toward injecting drug users and truckers produced by Sai Paranjpye are being shown widely in India and provide another unique opportunity for documenting and evaluating the effectiveness of such stigma reduction media products. Additionally, to promote greater use of these products as learning tools, viewer or listener guides could help increase understanding and discussion among audiences. These guides could be disseminated through networks and community organizations interested in hosting viewings or listening sessions.

Further Sharpen and Refine Tools for Religious Leaders

Relatively few stigma reduction efforts worldwide have involved religious leaders, yet their involvement presents a rich opportunity given their enormous reach and influence. Lessons from SARDM implementers' successes working with religious leaders, combined with existing tools and lessons in this area, could be a valuable resource in future efforts to engage religious leaders to address stigma and discrimination. The interventions, training tools, and other materials for religious leaders produced by Concern Worldwide, the Afghan Family Guidance Association, the Afghan Help and Training Program, and the

Voluntary Health Association of Tripura merit further attention and possibly development for broader use. The lessons from these efforts may be worth documenting for broader dissemination to other community organizations.

Foster Stronger Private Sector Engagement for Greater Economic Opportunity

Economic empowerment approaches, when implemented in conjunction with stigma reduction activities, have enormous promise for reducing stigma and discrimination experienced by marginalized populations and improving their health and well-being. Work with private sector partners, however, represents a gap in experience. Although many SARDM implementers established productive relationships with the government, efforts to engage the private sector were rare and fraught with challenge. In settings where employment opportunities are scarce, securing formal sector jobs for marginalized populations can be especially difficult. The time and effort involved for community organizations—especially small, relatively new groups—may not be cost-effective. A broader policy effort, such as advocacy with government to offer private sector incentives for hiring marginalized populations, could ease the way for community organizations running employment programs. Social enterprise efforts, such as the Ashodaya restaurant created by sex workers, showed promise and merit further exploration and investment.

Ensure That an Expanded Response to Stigma and Discrimination Provides Economic Opportunities for Marginalized Populations

A number of SARDM implementers hired and paid people from marginalized groups to help conduct project activities. This approach provided powerful benefits to participants, giving them new skills and self-confidence, and contributed to project success. As stigma reduction efforts expand, ensuring that organizations continue to hire people from marginalized groups as much as possible to implement work will be important. The income offers people multiple benefits and helps combat the perception that people from marginalized groups cannot be productive, valuable contributors to their families and communities.

Support Implementers in Strengthening Their Capacity to Expand

The efforts of SARDM implementers to address stigma and discrimination reflect a great deal of courage, commitment, and talent. These characteristics are fundamental for expansion. But if these groups are to lead substantially larger efforts, many will need capacity strengthening in areas such as programming strategies, management systems, and monitoring and evaluation. Producing effective tools and products, for example, can require a high degree of experience and skill. Materials must be carefully crafted and tested so that they further project goals and do not unintentionally reinforce stigma and harmful stereotypes. In addition, the capacity to monitor and assess progress is critical not only for promoting continued improvement, but also for making the case to donors and governments for program expansion and increased investment. As implementers seek to expand their work and procure new funding, being able to document how their stigma reduction interventions link to concrete outcomes in behavior change and service use will be increasingly important.

PART II

Six Case Studies Highlighting Best Practices for Reducing Stigma and Discrimination

The research team of the International Center for Research on Women analyzed six of the projects in depth. These projects were selected for their potential promise in terms of scale and effect, operational feasibility, and diversity in terms of populations served. Unfortunately, the research team was not able to visit all 26 implementers, especially because security concerns deter travel in some of the areas where implementers are working. The following case studies provide a closer look at how implementers in different settings formulated highly creative responses to stigma and discrimination. The projects were implemented by Job Opportunity and Business Support and Nari Unnayan Shakti in Bangladesh and by Lotus, Swathi Mahila Sanga, The Communication Hub, and We Care in India.

CHAPTER 6

Using Theater to Reduce Stigma and Discrimination against Men Who Have Sex with Men in Rural South India

In India, stigma and discrimination often prevent men who have sex with men (MSM) from accessing government entitlements or seeking justice for such abuses of their rights as police violence or refusal of health services. Their experience of stigma tends to be particularly severe because it stems not only from their perceived association with HIV but also from their sexuality.

Theater offers a strong mechanism for changing deep-seated cultural attitudes about gender and sexuality that drive stigma. More than a strictly informational intervention, theater has the potential to alter damaging but deeply entrenched social norms.

Lotus Integrated AIDS Awareness Sangam, founded in 2000, is a membership organization that supports MSM in Kumbakonam and surrounding villages in Tamil Nadu, India. Lotus works with about 1,500 members, organizing membership meetings, providing counseling, and undertaking advocacy efforts to reduce stigma and discrimination and prevent HIV transmission. Lotus, which is community run, is one of the few groups in India working with MSM in rural and semi-urban areas.

Lotus recognized the potential power of theater to promote positive social change. With its South Asia Region Development Marketplace (SARDM) grant, Lotus developed a theater program in and around its rural base in Tamil Nadu, India, aimed at changing harmful attitudes and practices preventing MSM and transgender persons from accessing legal redress through their municipal governments known as *panchayats*. Panchayats are powerful local bodies that regulate the sociopolitical norms at the village and semi-urban levels; they are the primary avenues through which citizens pursue justice at the village and semi-urban levels, even before engaging local police. Panchayat leaders are in a unique position to model new attitudes and behaviors for the broader community, setting an example that could enhance the quality of life and access to benefits and services among marginalized populations.

Lotus's play tells the story of a young man who has sex with men and whose parents are determined to get him married. It follows the protagonist, Ranjith, through daily life, depicting the stigma and discrimination he experiences at home, in his neighborhood, and from his friends. In one pivotal scene, Ranjith stands alone on the stage and expresses how what he experiences makes him feel, how much it hurts, and how he was born with feelings he cannot change. Crying out to God, he asks, "Why have you given me this life?" At that moment in the play, the audience always becomes silent and attentive. In another pivotal scene, the parents take Ranjith to meet his future bride and parents-in-law. The prospective bride, Susila, recognizes the situation and explains, "Your son is a man with a female heart." She refers the family to Lotus Sangam counseling, explaining that Lotus is a support organization for MSM and transgender persons. Susila also asks the father not to force his son into marriage, which would spoil the life of both his son and a potential bride. In the final scene, Ranjith and his parents visit the counselor at Lotus, who answers all of their questions. These questions clearly mirror those of the audience, because at this point they usually lean toward the stage in anticipation of the answers.

Implementation

Lotus used a careful process to develop and implement the theater intervention. They conducted focus group interviews with MSM and panchayat leaders to inform script development and provide baseline data for an evaluation. A member of Lotus wrote the script. The implementation process also involved hiring the project's staff, securing and setting up office and performance practice space, contracting professional theater trainers, and holding auditions for the performers who made up the theater troupe (which Lotus refers to as the "cultural team").

With core funding from SARDM, Lotus mobilized additional support from the Indian Network for People Living with HIV/AIDS to intensify its work with panchayat leaders in performance villages. This work entailed organizing two one-day trainings for panchayat leaders about HIV and AIDS, MSM, and transgender populations.

Lotus selected villages for the performances on the basis of the group's knowledge of where MSM resided and the willingness of panchayat leaders to have a performance in their community. Because Lotus had a letter of support from the Tamil Nadu State AIDS Control Society, its entry into villages was relatively smooth. In total, Lotus organized 75 performances of the play in three districts over the course of one year, reaching approximately 11,250 villagers. Lotus collected end-line data on the results in October and November 2009 and disseminated the findings in December 2009.

Results

The project successfully opened a justice channel through panchayat leaders and achieved an array of unanticipated outcomes. Panchayat leaders reported changes in their attitudes and behaviors, while MSM confirmed positive changes in their lives. The intervention also strengthened Lotus itself, improving its ability to use theater, improving the health and well-being of its members, and leading to mobilization of additional funds.

Changes at the Panchayat Level

Panchayat leaders described a change in their understanding of MSM and transgender individuals and the stigma and discrimination these individuals face. Leaders said that they anticipate this new understanding will change their future behavior toward MSM and transgender individuals:

> This was the first time I had understood that there are men who wear pants like men but feel like women inside. I only knew about transgender persons, men who wear women's clothes, but not about men who wear clothes like men but have a heart of a woman.

Panchayat leaders emphasized the following points that they and their village members learned through the play:

- MSM face stigma and discrimination in all areas of life:

  The play showed us how discrimination occurs by friends, families, and communities. The scene that really touched me was the one where the parents are shown harassing their son [a man who has sex with men]. It really hurts to see parents treating their own child like this. This was very painful to see.

- Forced marriages ruin the lives of MSM and the women they marry:

  By forcing MSM to marry, we are not solving any problem. It is not helping the MSM or the women they marry.

- Stigma and discrimination have severe consequences for MSM, including having to leave home and being denied employment opportunities. They are left with few survival options:

  I advise that the government should come forward for transgender persons and MSM so that they can get a job or employment, so they don't have to beg or [sell] sex just to live.

- MSM and transgender persons have talents and skills to contribute to and participate in family and community life.

  The play showed that they have very special talents and that they can live with a profession, that they don't have to just live by alms. They can be self-sufficient if they can live with self-esteem and contribute to society. I think that MSM should be treated equally and they should be given more skills and [a] trade so they can live independently and . . . with self-esteem.

Panchayat leaders also expressed an intention to intervene on behalf of MSM and transgender persons in instances of harassment and abuse. One leader said, "If I come to know of an MSM, I would refer him to Lotus. And if I see an MSM being teased, I would interfere [and] advise [the harassers] to stop and . . . not tease them."

Lotus members and MSM in the villages confirmed that many of the panchayat leaders were behaving differently toward them after seeing the play. They reported changes ranging from "He now greets me when he sees me" to "I am now treated with respect; he even invites me for tea and offers me a lift in his vehicle." The consensus among MSM interviewed was that although they thought all panchayat leaders had understood the issues presented in the play, about half had an exceptionally strong positive reaction. For example, some panchayat leaders are actively seeking out MSM under their jurisdiction to talk with them, to tell them about the play, and to encourage them to visit Lotus offices.

MSM also reported that panchayat leaders have intervened against the type of daily harassment that drives marginalized communities further underground and deters care seeking. A Lotus member mentioned this anecdote:

> One panchayat leader who saw the play, when he saw some boys harassing a group of transgenders begging for alms, . . . stopped his vehicle and told the boys to stop. He told the boys that transgenders are also human beings and deserve to be treated with the same respect as others.

Another Lotus member recalled being referred to Lotus by a panchayat leader:

> One day after the play, the panchayat leader came to me and asked me if I had contact with Lotus and why don't I get into contact with them, as I could get some benefits from that. . . . The leader is now very friendly, and when he sees me on the road, he gives me a lift and encourages me to go to Lotus. Before the play, this leader used to tease me, asking, "Should I call you a she or a he?" But since the play he now greets me, encourages me to seek out Lotus, and is nice to me.

Changes among Marginalized Populations

One of the challenges in meeting the needs of marginalized populations is that stigma and discrimination tend to reduce care seeking and health service use. MSM in the villages discussed how important the play was for them in recognizing that they were not alone, that others were like them, and that a support group existed that they could join. As a cultural team member explained, "I have recognized my own problems through this process. I have come to accept myself, know more about myself, and have a group to belong to. I am not feeling shy and ashamed anymore." As of mid-December 2009, 147 "hidden" MSM had approached the actors after a performance; of those, 47 visited Lotus offices, often at some distance from their villages, to seek support. Of the 47, 42 accessed counseling services at Lotus. Of those counseled, 19 were referred to the government hospital for testing for HIV and sexually transmitted infections and received treatment as needed.

Changes in Villagers' Behavior

The interviewed MSM described an array of improvements in their daily lives resulting from the play. After the performance, many reported a drop in harassment in public spaces, such as the market or taxi stands, as well as a new willingness by villagers to engage in normal daily social interactions with them. Some reported that villagers even apologized for their past behavior. Others reported how some villagers have stepped in to challenge teasing and harassment of MSM and transgender persons, something that never occurred before the play. For example, a cultural team member reported, "I was in the fish market, where I usually get teased and harassed. Suddenly one man, who had seen the play in his village, stood up and told the fishmongers they should stop the teasing. He explained about the play and the messages. I was so happy."

Moreover, these changes may be lasting. As one Lotus member reported, "Change is continuing. The play was about one year ago in my village. Till now the change has continued."

Organizational Strengthening for Lotus

The project's capacity-strengthening benefits are multiple. In general, the response to HIV stigma is inadequate, and efforts in this area led by marginalized communities themselves are especially scarce. Thus, the project served a critical organizational strengthening role for further larger-scale efforts. Lotus staff members have gained experience and skills in project management and implementation, including accounting, financial and technical reporting, monitoring and evaluation, event planning, training, and negotiating with panchayat leaders. They have also acquired capabilities in developing scripts, acting, and using street theater for effective messaging. As the director reported, "Now I can manage a project, and I can teach people how to manage a project. . . . I have learned about documentation, research, team management, [and] accounts management."

A number of organizational changes and new high-profile commitments have resulted from the theater project. Lotus is now a member of a national transgender convening committee supported by the United Nations Development Programme and has received support from the Indian Network for People Living with HIV/AIDS to conduct trainings and participate in local and state-level events, such as World AIDS Day. In addition, Lotus now participates in important meetings and events in Tamil Nadu on MSM and transgender persons. Lotus is also a founding community-based organization for a state-level forum, the United Network of MSM Advocacy and AIDS Initiatives (UNMAAI—in Tamil, this means truth or fact). At the local level, panchayats have invited Lotus representatives to attend village events to raise awareness about stigma toward MSM and transgender persons. Lotus has also received several international visitors seeking to learn more about the project and view a performance, and it was hired by an international researcher to conduct field interviews that culminated in January 2010.

The Lotus director sums up the positive influence of the project as follows, in terms of both organizational strengthening and the new respect others have for his organization as a result of the intervention:

> Before this project, people didn't believe Lotus had the capacity to implement projects. We proved through this project we can implement projects and through the cultural team that we have the capacity to communicate messages in a good way and the courage to communicate things that are very sensitive.

Lessons Learned

The success of Lotus's project in reducing stigma and discrimination toward and among MSM and transgender persons comes from the confluence of several key factors:

- *Staff commitment.* Lotus staff and cultural team members exhibited extraordinary determination, courage, and dedication in addressing sensitive issues in the public forum of theater. The power of the collective voice and the safety net of a close-knit group to support and care for the members have proved critical to the success of this process.
- *Theater as a medium for change.* Theater creates a unique space to address sensitive and taboo topics that could not otherwise be discussed publicly in a mixed forum of women and men and across generations. Furthermore, in putting these issues out in the open, plays create a new space for discussion and action.
- *Carefully targeted messaging.* Skillful communication, careful crafting of messages, and clever use of street theater were all keys to the project's success. The play was simultaneously entertaining and educational. It held the audience's attention and appealed to people's emotions and better instincts. Finally, it successfully conveyed several key messages about what it means to be a man who has sex with men or a transgender person and the need to adopt more positive attitudes and behaviors toward these marginalized groups.
- *Skillful and heartfelt theater performances.* Audience members felt and understood that although the performance was a play, it was depicting the real, lived experiences of the actors. Linked to this understanding

was the opportunity for the village audience to develop empathy for individual team members and their characters. Before and after the performance, villagers could ask questions and approach members of the performance team and Lotus staff individually. In addition, before each performance, each audience member received a flyer that described what the play would be about and Lotus's contact information.

CHAPTER 7

Fighting Internalized Stigma among Injecting Drug Users in Bangladesh: A Combination Program to Support Economic and Social Reintegration

Injecting drug users (IDUs) leaving drug rehabilitation centers in Bangladesh face multiple challenges managing their drug use or staying drug free and reintegrating into their families and society. These challenges are compounded by their inability to find employment and overcome the stigma and discrimination they face as former IDUs. Their low self-esteem and lack of basic education and vocational skills, as well as the scarcity of jobs in general in Bangladesh, make finding gainful employment and reentering the workforce even more difficult for former IDUs.

Job Opportunity and Business Support (JOBS), established in 1997, is a nonprofit organization based in Dhaka that aims to combat economic discrimination against the underprivileged in Bangladesh by creating enterprises and jobs. Since 2006, JOBS has been working with former IDUs, rehabilitation centers, and the private sector in Bangladesh to enhance reintegration of former IDUs into economic and social life.

As a South Asia Regional Development Marketplace (SARDM) grant recipient, JOBS expanded its job skills training program to include a stigma reduction component for IDUs. The SARDM-funded project had two goals:

- To provide former male IDUs with economic opportunities and to facilitate their road to economic independence so that they could regain their self-esteem and dignity as productive members of society
- To facilitate reconnection with family members, help participants overcome internalized stigma, and raise awareness to fight HIV stigma and discrimination among the general public.

Male IDUs were included in this project because they are considered the highest-risk population and most vulnerable to HIV.

Implementation

JOBS worked closely with rehabilitation centers in Dhaka to select former male IDUs for specialized job training coupled with a stigma reduction component. Of 52 former IDUs interviewed, 20 participants were selected on the basis of factors such as history of past drug use and violence on the job. JOBS staff then arranged with Fibertech mannequin company to hire former IDUs for factory work and begin a new production line. JOBS subsidized the former IDUs' salaries for the first three months of the project with the agreement that if workers achieved the technical skills and productivity expected by the end of the probation period, the firm would hire them. As part of the project's stigma reduction component, the former IDUs produced 50 red mannequins and designed clothes with the AIDS ribbon to be used in advocacy efforts throughout Dhaka. JOBS also assigned two dedicated staff members, who provided informal counseling to participants for the first six months and coordinated weekly visits from a rehabilitation center counselor.

To decrease the likelihood of relapse, the work site for mannequin production was located in a part of Dhaka removed from the participants' existing environment (including friends and family), and living quarters were provided on site. This strategy limited the environmental cues that might tempt participants to use drugs and had the added benefit of moving participants to a community in which their history of drug use was unknown. To foster peer support and help prevent relapse, the production unit employed the former IDUs as a group. Participants within such groups included a mix of men recently out of rehabilitation centers and men out for longer periods of time, an arrangement that encouraged a supportive environment.

Before working at the factory, participants completed a five-day course using the Workplace Discipline and Congenial Environment (WDCE) curriculum. This training aimed to provide individuals with the requisite skills to be successful in a factory environment and a basic understanding of financial management to prepare them for economic independence. A combination of didactic and participatory methods was used along with confidence-building exercises. Following the WDCE training, participants received hands-on instruction in the production of mannequins. Last, a focus group discussion was conducted to provide participants with information about HIV prevention and transmission and to dispel misconceptions.

The first month of the training program was a grace period to allow participants to adjust to their new environment and work life. The grace period proved challenging, and participants needed regular support and encouragement from the JOBS team. However, by the end of the second month, participation and focus had improved greatly, overtime increased, and attendance improved. At the completion of the six-month training program, the 50 red mannequins required for the stigma reduction component of the project had been completed.

In the second stage of the project, seven of the men who performed well during the first six months were selected for additional block-batik training to design clothes with red ribbons. These clothes would then be displayed on the red mannequins developed by the former IDUs as part of an advocacy campaign.

In the final stage of the project, an advocacy campaign was undertaken in well-known stores throughout Dhaka, with strong support from boutique owners and local fashion designers and from Bibi Russell, the United Nations ambassador for HIV and AIDS. At each store, a red mannequin wearing white clothes with red ribbon designs produced by the former IDUs was displayed alongside information on the project and on HIV, injecting drug use, and stigma and discrimination in Bangladesh. Information was provided in English and Bengali. JOBS provided store owners with basic information about HIV and the project so they could respond to customers' questions. Mannequins and advocacy materials were also displayed at drug rehabilitation centers, social clubs, and hotels. They also were included in workshops for university students, and an article about the project was published in a magazine.

Results

Overall, the job-training and confidence-building component was a success. Of participants trained and employed through the program, 75 percent were accepted back into their families by the end of the project period. This acceptance was linked to their success in regaining trust by staying away from drugs and to their ability to hold a steady job and save money to contribute to the family income again. The fact that participants maintained employment and reintegrated into family life after the program ended indicates that negative attitudes about former IDUs among employers and family members can shift with a combination of job-training and confidence-building interventions. Job-training and confidence-building efforts also helped participants overcome the internal stigma that kept them from succeeding in the past. Such efforts enabled participants to demonstrate that they could be productive members of society again. However, as one former IDU said, "Recovery starts from the rehab but doesn't end there. Society has a huge role to play."

In addition, participants learned important information about HIV and AIDS. Many were confident enough to share this information with other current and former drug users. One former IDU explained:

> Since I joined the JOBS project, I have been away from drugs. I also learned a lot about HIV and gained some technical skills. I am now very careful in my sex life. I inform other drug users about HIV and how to protect themselves. . . . I tell them to spend Tk 3 to buy clean needles instead of sharing. I also tell them about using condoms during sex.

Of the 20 participants trained, two started their own business selling daily items, five moved to jobs with better salaries, six shifted to another factory that opened, and six were offered alternative job opportunities but opted to pursue their own interests and leads. Only one participant dropped out. A former IDU expressed his appreciation of the program:

> The skills and employment have led to better behavior ... and made my life beautiful.

A mannequin production trainer found that families were also appreciative:

> The families of the participants were very happy to see them working and would often ask me to please look after their son and keep him away from drugs.

The block-batik trainer explained how the job skills training empowered participants and built confidence in their creative abilities:

[The men] were very motivated and had a sense of pride at being able to create something. [The block-batik training] empowered them, as they got to decide what size the AIDS ribbon should be for the various garments, what the placement of the ribbons and design should be, etc. It was important for me to respect their opinions.

The snowball effect of the project at the rehabilitation center was impressive. The rehabilitation center staff noted that the number of requests to enroll in the rehabilitation program nearly doubled as IDUs learned of the JOBS training program.

Participants and program managers alike thought the advocacy component could have been expanded. Although the red mannequins succeeded in attracting attention, how effective this strategy was in changing negative attitudes toward former IDUs remains unclear. The shops that participated in the advocacy campaign were mainly high end. Shop owners noted that few people asked questions about the project or the information presented. Former IDUs suggested that in the future the campaign should be expanded to include shops catering to a wider spectrum of society. In addition, as noted by the block-batik trainer, the former IDUs would have appreciated the opportunity to be more involved in advocacy and outreach efforts:

The men appreciated the advocacy objective of the project and having a hand in it. They even wanted to make their own t-shirts with the AIDS ribbon. I was surprised and asked if they would really wear them. They said they would wear them because they wanted to be able to do advocacy on their own.

A former IDU explained why the men wanted to participate in outreach efforts:

We want the next generation of IDUs to be assisted and not to be looked at as people who only deserve to be hated.

Lessons Learned

A key lesson of this project was the importance of using a combination of approaches to build self-confidence and challenge internalized stigma to enable economic and social reintegration. The experiences of the IDUs reinforce the widely accepted notion that having economic independence and being a productive member of society provide the basic foundation for regaining self-confidence and obtaining the strength to avoid relapse. The success of the JOBS project suggests that programs targeting IDUs for stigma reduction need to combine drug and economic rehabilitation with counseling and skills building.

Another lesson was the importance of involving well-trained, sincere, and committed counselors to support and respond to the complex needs of the former IDUs immediately following their relocation. The quality of counseling that the rehabilitation center staff provided proved to be insufficient and needed to be supplemented with support from the JOBS staff. Future projects should identify counselors with proper qualifications and "soft skills" (being compassionate, caring, supportive, and so on) and should consider training former IDUs to be mentors and assist in peer counseling.

JOBS staff members interacted with sincerity and provided continuous reassurance to the participants throughout the duration of the project. Most participants had extremely low self-esteem, having been isolated from their families and society for a long period because of their drug use. The compassion of JOBS staff members encouraged former IDUs to share their concerns and challenges, which enabled JOBS to respond immediately and identify solutions to their complex needs. This personal interaction also expedited the social reintegration process and assisted former IDUs in regaining self-confidence and basic social skills. In addition, JOBS staff members found that supporting the former IDUs' ideas, listening to their suggestions, and recognizing their achievements with training completion certificates and consistent positive reinforcement were critical for building self-esteem and self-confidence and keeping the men actively engaged in the project.

Finally, the sustainability of job skills and employment support projects for IDUs is clearly a challenge. At the start of the project, the private sector partner initially identified was reluctant to commit to investing in and starting a new product unit, so JOBS had to identify a new partner. However, the partner company sold the mannequin production unit after the project ended, which meant that several participants lost their jobs. Identifying placement opportunities where former IDUs can learn general, readily transferrable skills, rather than specialized skills, is optimal. However, the support of the private sector partners' management, working, and living environments is equally important, and such support should be taken into account when considering employment options and business partners.

Although providing salaries and counseling support to former IDUs for the first three months of the project helped enhance physical, social, and economic rehabilitation, both participants and project staff members noted that extending this support for six months would have been better. Such support would encourage more private sector firms to become involved in economic rehabilitation programs for former IDUs, giving the former IDUs more job options to choose from. Organizations wishing to replicate this project should bear in mind the intensive support required in the first six months for this type of intervention to be successful.

CHAPTER 8

The Gateway to Public Opinion: Harnessing Local Journalists to Fight Stigma and Discrimination in Bangladesh

The media have a critical role to play in reducing HIV stigma and discrimination. Yet the language and images portrayed in print and broadcast media often unintentionally foster stigma and discrimination toward people living with HIV and groups considered particularly vulnerable to HIV infection. In an effort to ensure that journalists in Bangladesh were fighting stigma instead of propagating it, Nari Unnayan Shakti (NUS)[1] conducted a countrywide training program to increase in-depth knowledge and understanding of HIV and stigma and discrimination and to enhance journalists' skills in articulating this information in newspaper articles.

Established in 1992, NUS is a nonprofit organization that aims at bringing positive changes to the women and children of Bangladesh in a number of critical development areas. NUS has been involved in HIV prevention, care, and support activities since 1993 and began working to reduce stigma and discrimination in 2005 by organizing a regional meeting on the issue in collaboration with the Commonwealth of Asia Center. As a South Asia Region Development Marketplace grant recipient, NUS expanded its stigma reduction efforts to include the media. By working with local newspaper journalists, editors, and newspaper owners, NUS supported the publication of articles and reports on HIV, AIDS, and HIV-related stigma and discrimination in numerous dailies across Bangladesh.

Implementation

This project included a series of trainings for journalists related to how they portray HIV and stigma, followed by a competition for best articles on the topic. The project targeted local journalists for these trainings because the project team felt they would have more influence with local opinion leaders than would national journalists. During the project's first four months, NUS gained the necessary clearance from the government to conduct the trainings and adapted relevant training materials for the Bangladesh context. These materials consisted of sessions on the epidemiology of HIV, on understanding and challenging HIV stigma and discrimination, and on nonstigmatizing language and messaging. NUS also reprinted two Bengali booklets on HIV for trainees. NUS then sent expression of interest letters regarding the project to all registered, high-circulation daily newspapers in the country.[2] Seventy percent of the dailies contacted responded. NUS then followed up directly with editors to ensure that they sent properly trained, competent journalists to participate in the training. The editors were also expected to provide space for publishing articles on HIV, AIDS, and stigma.

Beginning in November 2008, NUS organized six trainings of two days' duration throughout the country. The trainings covered all 64 districts. They were participatory and included interaction and discussion with people living with HIV. Participants had time to draft articles and receive critical feedback from senior journalists and editors. Each training began with a two-hour inaugural session, to which key stakeholders—including senior government officials, the police superintendent, the president of the local press club, civil society representatives, the program manager of the National AIDS/Sexually Transmitted Disease Programme, the Joint Secretary of Health and Family Welfare, and the press—were invited. During this session, presentations were given on the HIV epidemic in Bangladesh and the challenges posed by stigma and discrimination. Overall, 288 journalists and other stakeholders participated in the inaugural sessions for the six trainings, and 137 local journalists were trained.

Following the training, participants were asked to submit copies of articles they had written about HIV, AIDS, and stigma and discrimination as well as articles they had published. NUS followed up with journalists to encourage article submission and, as an incentive, provided certificates to those who submitted articles. The articles were then entered in a competition. The top three stories were selected on the basis of article structure, factual content, and appropriate discussion of stigma in the context of HIV. Senior media representatives, including the head of a national television station and two editors of national newspapers, judged the competition. The winners were recognized in an awards ceremony on World AIDS Day at the culmination of the project.

Results

The project succeeded at helping local journalists channel their new understanding about HIV and stigma into articles that were then published throughout Bangladesh. By the end of the project period, 78 (57 percent) of the journalists trained had published related articles in their local papers.

Participants clearly benefited from and appreciated the participatory training method. As one male journalist noted:

> The most impressive thing about the training was that it was participatory; we learned by doing. This is unique; I have never been to a workshop like that before. Whatever we were taught, we had to practice during the training.

The participation of people living with HIV in the training proved especially powerful for journalists. According to the project director, many of the journalists had never met a person living with HIV. Interacting with people living with HIV allowed the journalists to overcome their own fears and misconceptions and helped them understand the stigma and discrimination that people living with HIV face. This experience equipped the journalists to better address stigma and discrimination in their writings.

The interaction was also beneficial for the people living with HIV who participated and the networks for HIV-positive people they represented. The training provided an opportunity for the networks in three regions to link with the media and the local administration, which project sponsors hope will lead to more strategic engagement with local government and the media.

The involvement of key stakeholders, such as national and local government officials, police officers, and members of civil society, from the onset of the project and in the inaugural events also contributed to the success of the project. Having clear support from senior-level government officials added credibility to the trainings, which in turn helped draw journalists from high-circulation dailies to the training and attracted more press coverage. For example, after the initial inaugural session, all of the high-circulation newspapers in Bangladesh published one article on the project itself, and 11 television stations ran a story about the project. As one senior government official noted, "It gives the project more weight to know that national commitment is there, [that] it's not just a [non-governmental organization] running a project." Involving these stakeholders also expanded the reach of stigma reduction efforts in other key sectors with influence over the treatment of people living with HIV. During the training, many of these stakeholders—such as local government officials and police officers—committed to support people living with HIV.

Another important factor contributing to the high number of articles published after the trainings was the considerable follow-up NUS conducted both with training participants to encourage article submission and with editors to encourage publication. The project director noted that of the 78 journalists who submitted articles, only 60 percent did so without being reminded. The level of follow-up needed is certainly a factor to be considered when planning media sensitization and training interventions.

Following the trainings, journalists were eager to continue learning from and sharing information with their colleagues about HIV, AIDS, and stigma and discrimination. Therefore, journalists, networks of people living with HIV, and NUS worked together to develop a national stigma reduction network. Participants were eager to continue this and other networking activities after the project ended; however, such activities will be contingent on the ability to secure additional funding. Support for such a network appears to exist in the national government, as noted by this Ministry of Health official: "It would be great to have a network of journalists trained on stigma and discrimination to make sure they remain engaged in the issue and continue to strengthen their capacity."

Lessons Learned

A number of important lessons from this project can help inform the expansion and replication of stigma reduction trainings for members of the media in Bangladesh and elsewhere. Both the government officials and senior media representatives interviewed appreciated the focus of the project on local journalists, who they felt have more influence with local opinion leaders than national journalists. However, many of these local journalists—especially in rural areas—lacked formal journalism training and experience. This gap was evident to the judges who selected the winning articles. Two of the judges interviewed noted that the quality of the writing, in terms of structure and language, could be improved, but they recognized that this improvement was not feasible with the current project structure, which did not include this type of capacity strengthening. To address this gap, they suggested offering follow-up refresher trainings combined with mentorships with senior journalists, who could critique articles and provide support as needed. The need for continued support was also reflected in the multiple requests for additional training.

The judges, as well as one of the journalists who participated in the training, also suggested that the project consider including broadcast (radio and television) journalists in trainings to expand the reach of media-focused stigma reduction efforts. These media channels are particularly important in Bangladesh, where the literacy rate is quite low and thus print media reaches only a limited segment of the population. Other stakeholders similarly noted that complementing stigma reduction training for the media with television and radio broadcasts of national information, education, and awareness campaigns on stigma and discrimination would be beneficial.

In terms of the training content, several government officials and senior media representatives interviewed suggested that it be expanded to include broader human rights issues, such as violence against women and human trafficking, as well as information on other important diseases. As one Ministry of Health official noted, "HIV is really a small issue in Bangladesh compared to some others." However, some of the participants said making the course longer would be difficult because of their time constraints. Instead, they suggested having refresher courses every few months. Organizations planning to implement media trainings should keep these points in mind and perhaps arrange a series of short trainings covering technical capacity building in relation to a range of human rights topics.

Some participants requested more in-depth knowledge on HIV to help them articulate the facts in their writing. As one female journalist said, "Once something is written, it holds more weight. So the writer needs to know and fully understand the topic." However, although providing detailed information about HIV is important, ensuring that journalists can address stigma and discrimination in the context of HIV in their articles is also critical. One of the challenges noted by project staff members and competition judges was that many of the articles written by trainees focused solely on HIV transmission and prevention with no discussion of stigma and discrimination. Trainees also tended to focus on sexual transmission rather than other modes of HIV transmission, such as needle sharing, that are common in Bangladesh. This omission further demonstrates that local journalists need additional training and follow-up to ensure full understanding of the biological and social aspects of HIV.

Another key lesson of this project was that good training materials for addressing stigma and discrimination exist and can be adapted relatively quickly to a particular audience, such as journalists. By adapting existing training materials and reprinting relevant factual booklets for participants, projects can conserve resources and expand the number of people reached through training and follow-up. Last, to enhance the effectiveness of HIV stigma reduction in Bangladesh, presenting HIV as a social issue rather than a health issue was suggested. As articulated by the editor of a national newspaper:

> HIV should not just be reported on the health page. It has to be addressed as a social issue, not a health issue, if you want to reduce stigma and remove the stereotypes and prejudice preexisting in society.

Notes

1. Nari Unnayan Shakti means women's power for development in Bengali.
2. High-circulation papers were those with a daily circulation of 10,000 or more subscribers.

CHAPTER 9

Taking It to the Village: Reducing Stigma through Traditional Street Theater in Tamil Nadu

In a village in Kancheepuram district, India, the narrator of a street theater performance tells the audience how, after testing positive for HIV, he was no longer allowed to eat with his siblings, he was scolded when he fell ill, and no one would touch his clothes, even though he and his brother used to wear each other's shirts.

The play was developed by We Care Social Service Society, a nongovernmental organization established in 1994 that runs a care facility for people living with HIV who have been abandoned or who are too sick to remain at home. We Care's services include nutritional, psychosocial, treatment adherence, and income-generating outreach support for people living with HIV. Because stigma and discrimination often hamper delivery of services, We Care applied to the South Asia Region Development Marketplace (SARDM) for a grant to use a traditional Tamilian street drama (*therukoothu*) to educate and promote discussion about HIV and its associated stigma and discrimination.

We Care's play stops at various points to allow villagers to ask questions about HIV and to discuss the storyline with members of the theater troupe, many of whom are living with HIV. The questions the villagers most commonly ask reflect their fears and misconceptions about HIV transmission:

- If a mosquito bites a person living with HIV and then bites another person, will it transmit HIV?
- If my HIV-positive brother wears my shirt, will it infect me through his sweat?
- If HIV can spread through blood, breast milk, and semen, why not through vomit?
- Can I buy vegetables from a woman living with HIV even if she touches the vegetables with her hand?
- Can we eat food cooked by a person living with HIV?

Fear of casual transmission is an important driver of HIV stigma and discrimination. It leads people to take what they believe are protective measures against HIV, such as isolating and avoiding people living with HIV. By having people living with HIV share their experiences and knowledge, the play conveys how these actions are hurtful and unnecessary. The storyline emphasizes key messages about HIV:

- HIV does not spread through casual contact, so one need not fear and isolate people living with HIV.
- People living with HIV can lead normal, long, healthy lives.
- A woman with HIV can have a child without HIV.

Actors living with HIV share testimonials, such as how care given by family members has enabled them to lead healthy lives and to support their families. These testimonies showcase to audiences supportive attitudes and behaviors.

Implementation

The troupe performed the play for three consecutive nights in each of 10 villages in Kancheepuram district. The play stopped at various points for discussion and information exchange with audience members. The troupe encouraged audience members to ask questions, offering prizes for participation. The troupe stayed in each village four days, allowing opportunities for interacting with village members and providing information about and referrals for voluntary counseling and testing and care services.

The project undertook a range of activities to develop and produce the play:

- *Script development.* A professional scriptwriter developed an initial storyline, and the HIV and stigma themes were added through a script development workshop that included people living with HIV, HIV experts, troupe members, and theater professionals. In the workshop, the team drew on data from interviews with people living with HIV from three networks in the district. The script combined well-known traditional, mythical stories with real-life experiences of people living with HIV, moving between the two and drawing parallels between modern life with HIV and the ancient stories. During the play, a narrator (*kattiakkaran*) would weave the past and present storylines together. The script continued to evolve throughout the training process and performances, integrating new ideas brought forward by the theater troupe as the process of performing unfolded and taking into account audience questions and reactions.

- *Selection and training of the theater troupe.* Although the original idea had been that the troupe would consist only of people living with HIV (nonprofessional actors), the impracticality of this scheme quickly became apparent. Therefore, the project formed a mixed troupe of professional and nonprofessional actors, which ended up providing opportunities for stigma reduction among the HIV-negative performers. The performance team consisted of seven professional theater performers, five nonprofessional performers living with HIV, and three HIV-negative nonprofessional volunteers. The performers were trained for two months in an array of issues, including self-esteem, group dynamics, team building, life skills, appropriate ways to present themselves in the villages, script development, and *therukoothu*-style performance.

- *Selection of villages and the village project support committees.* With the help of the Tamil Nadu Network for Positive Persons, the project team identified 10 villages that had at least four people living with HIV and in which stigma was particularly problematic. Key leaders in each of these villages, including leaders from youth and women's groups, were contacted and invited to form project support committees. These committees took full ownership of the program. At their own expense, they organized boarding and lodging for the troupe, arranged a stage and sound system for the performance, and generated publicity about the event in the community.

Results

The project results indicate benefits to multiple stakeholders, including troupe members, villagers, and people living with HIV, though estimating the benefits to this last group was more difficult because many people fear stigma and discrimination and are not open about their status.

Effect on Troupe Members

Evidence suggests the play empowered troupe members living with HIV, as one man, an actor in the play, recounted:

> When I am providing the information [in the play], it makes me feel stronger. . . . I am telling people they can live long with HIV if they take medicine, and so that reinforces that [message] for me and encourages me to [take my medicine]. When I disclose my status on stage, afterwards it leads to [people living with HIV] coming to talk to me, and I can help them with information and referral to services like We Care. I also feel good to share that I got infected through sharing needles and that when I was doing this I did not know it could bring HIV. By sharing this information, hopefully I can prevent others getting infected this way.

The process of the training, performing, and belonging to an accepting, caring, and supportive group was life transforming for several of the troupe members living with HIV. It brought them not only new skills in theater, but also life and social skills that helped them integrate better in their communities and families. Most important, it built their self-esteem and confidence. For some, it provided the impetus and strength to reduce drug use. It also provided income, thereby allowing them to contribute to the household, and thus improved their status and reduced stigma at home. The same troupe member explained the significant positive influence his participation has had on his life:

> I credit this play with helping me to stop using drugs. I also learned how to take care of myself, [to] eat better.... When I was a drug addict, I used to think I was useless, . . . and I thought I should just use more drugs and die soon. But through the play I got . . . a reason to live, and so I stopped. Once I . . . decided to postpone my drug use, my life system changed. I no longer needed to steal to get money to get drugs—and now I can even save a little money and give [it] to my family.

Benefits extended to troupe members who are not living with HIV. One troupe member described the process of overcoming fear of contracting HIV through casual contact:

> We were very hesitant, afraid we would get infected from the [people living with HIV] in the group, at the beginning. . . . [W]e thought by eating from the same plate, touching, we could get HIV. The trainer and madam had to counsel us and explain that [HIV] could not spread this way. So from counseling we got over this, but it took some of us one month to stop asking for a separate plate. Now we are comfortable; we eat together, sleep together, bathe from the same pond, with no fears.

The project also built troupe members' skills and confidence to share information on HIV and challenge stigma in their own families and communities. As one member explained, "Some of the performances were held in our home villages, and we are now seen as a resource in those villages. People come to us to ask questions and for help." The professional troupe members are now, on their own time, taking the message and information they learned to schools.

Effect on Villagers

The play was well received in most villages, and evidence suggests villagers who attended the performances reflected on and shared the play's key messages. The size of the audience increased from one day to the next, indicating positive word of mouth about the play. One woman said, "It was so good we even missed our TV serials for this play. For three days we missed our serials." Interviews with a wide range of village members indicate that a key benefit of the play was that it opened space for and legitimized discussion of HIV (a taboo topic before the play), particularly between generations. As one woman explained, "Now we can tell, explain, and talk about HIV, which we could not do before—because it was thought to be such a dreaded disease." Village gatekeepers discussed how hesitant they had been at the beginning to allow the play to run because of the topic, but how happy they were that they had finally agreed.

Villagers were grateful to receive new information on HIV, especially about how it is and is not transmitted. They appreciated knowing that HIV cannot be transmitted through routine, daily contact. Many spoke of the fears they had prior to the play about contracting HIV through casual means and how this fear led them to discriminate against people living with HIV.

A number of villagers had not known that treatment for HIV existed or about the prevention of mother-to-child transmission. The fact that people living with HIV can live long and healthy lives and continue to contribute to their families and communities was also a new concept. Echoing a repeated sentiment, one woman explained that she had learned "that it is possible for [people living with HIV] to get married to each other and to live positively . . . and [t]hat we should not feel bad about HIV." The message about positive living came through in several scenes in the play, but troupe members who disclosed that they are living with HIV and talked about their own lives were able to deliver the message most compellingly. One group of young men said that the play has made them want to get tested for HIV, and they think it would be good if, in the future, HIV testing could be provided in conjunction with the performances.

The messages about the presence of stigma and discrimination and its effects on the lives of people living with HIV and their families were clearly heard and understood. Villagers described how stigma can lead to social and physical isolation and depression, can discourage people from taking medicine, and in extreme cases can result in suicide. At the end of one interview, an elderly woman confided that "long back there was a death here. He committed suicide because no one was accepting him, only his mother. Now we are aware and will not do such a thing again." Villagers, including children, also articulated specific stigmatizing behaviors that need to change in the community, explaining, "We should not keep away, we should not say 'don't sit with us, or eat with us.'. . . We know now that we can eat with them, share a dress with them, be in the same class."

Effect on People Living with HIV in Villages

Many people living with HIV in villages where the plays were performed have not disclosed their status publicly and therefore have not overtly experienced stigma and discrimination. But the play offered them a sense of hope about their prospects and reduced their fears of public disclosure. As one woman explained:

> Before I was afraid the general community people would stigmatize me if they got to know my status. Now, because of the play, I am less afraid of what might happen. . . . I [used to] worry for my son, that people will stop letting him play with their children if they find out he is HIV positive, but now I think, after the play, that might not be the case anymore.

People living with HIV also expressed that the play gave them strength. One woman living with HIV concluded, "These kinds of plays should be performed in many places as [people living with HIV] will get strength and support from it, and those who are negative will know how to prevent it."

Lessons Learned

Several important lessons for implementing drama-based stigma reduction interventions were learned from this project.

Patience and Persistence Are Key

A key lesson throughout the production process was the need for patience and persistence. The original plan had been to use only performers living with HIV, but the need for some professional troupe members, particularly musicians, became immediately apparent. The project found musicians, but they were reluctant to commit when they learned that they would be working with people living with HIV for fear of getting infected. They were eventually convinced to stay, but the process did take time and effort. Another challenge was finding people living with HIV who were willing to be trained as performers and travel to villages and who also could act, sing, and dance. The project had no success recruiting women living with HIV, and several of the men with HIV were drug users, posing challenges when relapses occurred and members could not work.

Patience and persistence were also needed to convince village gatekeepers to allow the play in their locale. Leaders in many villages were initially hesitant because of the topic. However, when a few performances had been held and word spread about how good the play was, villages began calling up to ask for performances. Unfortunately, We Care was not able to respond to this demand because the maximum number of villages feasible with the SARDM budget had already been selected.

Theater Has the Power to Open Discussion on Sensitive Topics among Diverse Audiences

A key finding of this intervention was that theater, which is viewed as nonthreatening and socially acceptable, is a powerful forum for broaching sensitive and taboo topics. It also is an ideal medium for allowing the same message to be heard by an audience diverse in both sex and age. That said, a well-crafted script that presents the sensitive issues and facts in an acceptable manner is crucial. The project struggled to find this balance at the beginning; some of the messages were too direct in the initial performances, leading to a negative response. By the fifth performance, the team used a more nuanced approach to convey sensitive information, such as the need to use condoms when having multiple partners.

Finding the Right Balance between Information and Entertainment Is a Process

Another challenge was striking the right balance between entertaining, which is necessary to hold the audience's attention, and delivering messages. The script continually evolved, sharpened through repeated performances and audience feedback. The performances gained strength as the project deepened its knowledge of audiences and crafted messages that responded specifically to knowledge gaps and transmission fears. The story also tapped the audience's basic desire to help, not harm, family and community members. The use of stop-start drama, where the play is stopped for interaction with the audience, was also an effective strategy for conveying information while sustaining the audience's attention.

Participation of People Living with HIV in Performances Is Critical to Audience Response

Knowing that some of the actors were living with HIV had a powerful effect on audiences. This factor intensified the messages delivered during performances. After seeing the play, villagers talked about how they had not realized what stigma and discrimination did and how they now understood and would no longer practice stigma and discrimination. They also talked at length about the importance of supporting people living with HIV so that such people can lead a healthy and productive life.

Village Participation Was a Key Factor in Success

Another key to success was creating ownership among people in the villages. In each village, for example, volunteers served on village committees that raised funds to house and feed the theater troupe for three nights, procured equipment and space, printed flyers, and generated publicity for the show. The presence of the theater troupe in the village was also important. Villagers conversed with troupe members during the day, asking questions and, in some cases, seeking care and service referrals. These interactions also allowed the troupe to alter the performance to respond to specific questions raised during the day.

Postproject Demand Remains Strong

Even after the project ended, demand for the play has continued to grow. Other villages have been calling to request performances, two local corporations have sponsored performances in additional villages (beyond what was possible in the SARDM budget), and the United Nations Children's Fund has asked We Care to submit a proposal to conduct the play in more villages. The play has created the roots of change in the villages where it was performed; however, as one of the directors of We Care pointed out, "Change takes time and requires ongoing support." Village leaders and members echoed this sentiment, stating that they would like—and needed—the play to return again to their village to make sure the message is heard by all.

CHAPTER 10

Celebrating Those Who Care: A Radio Program by HIV-Positive Journalists in Maharashtra

> To be frank, when I first came to know [about the possibility of doing an interview], I was scared, but then I thought . . . if by telling my story I can reach all people in Maharashtra, this will help reduce stigma, and so I should do it. And those who are negative will begin to think that they need to help people living with HIV, like my friend Arun has done, and this will help to reduce stigma. I got the very great opportunity; I can reach many people with my story and reduce stigma; it makes me feel good.
>
> —Project participant, The Communication Hub

Worldwide, most care for people living with HIV is provided not through health institutions but by family and, in some cases, friends. Although outright desertion by family is relatively rare, many people living with HIV experience isolation and neglect, which adversely affects their health and quality of life. Even so, some individuals, despite society's negative attitudes, provide care and support to people living with HIV on a daily basis. Yet their stories are rarely heard.

The Communication Hub (TCH), formed in 2007, harnesses communication to address a wide range of health and development issues, such as HIV and AIDS, reproductive health and sexuality, polio, tuberculosis, and sanitation. Using South Asia Regional Development

Marketplace grant money, TCH partnered with the Network of Maharashtra People Living with HIV (NMP+), which is now present in 26 districts in the state, to develop a 13-part radio serial to highlight the stories of people living with HIV and a significant person in their life who supports them.

"We wanted to talk about them, share their stories, listen to them, get inspired by them, celebrate them," explained Sonalini Mirchandani, the chief executive of TCH. The project, by showcasing individuals from all walks of life who support people living with HIV, communicates to the radio listener what nonstigmatizing and nondiscriminatory behavior is and aims to inspire audiences to emulate this behavior. See, for example, box 10.1.

In weaving these stories into a serial, the team includes critical information on HIV and AIDS. The serial addresses misconceptions about HIV and people living with HIV and provides a means for the radio audience members to act on what they have heard. Episodes include information on available testing, care, and treatment services, as well as contact information for NMP+.

Because the radio serial has not yet been broadcast as of the publication date of this case study, the following sections describe the implementation process and the lessons and results connected with this process. The Maharashtra State AIDS Control Society—supported by the National AIDS Control Organisation—has recently included the program in its next financial year media budget (April 2010–March 2011),

---

Box 10.1

Radio Episode Highlighting the Importance of Networks of People Living with HIV

Aruna, whose baby died of AIDS, discovered after her child's death that both she and her husband were living with HIV. Her husband died soon after, and Aruna was alone. However, her parents supported her and encouraged her to take up some work. Support from her colleagues, and later from a counselor from NMP+, helped bring Aruna back from a state of complete despair to a new life. She resumed her education and joined the network to become an active member, determined that others should not have to face the despair and fear that she went through.

Source: The Communicatiion Hub.

so the project team anticipates the serial will be broadcast over the next year.

Implementation

With rural Maharashtra as the target, the project team opted to use radio for several reasons. Radio is relatively low cost and reaches a large audience. Listeners may not have access to electricity or television, may be mobile, or may have low literacy. The project is planning to broadcast the series through India's public station, All India Radio, which has near universal reach in Maharashtra. Its 20 stations in Maharashtra reach a population of approximately 96.9 million, including about 55.8 million people residing in rural areas. In addition, as the project team noted, "Radio has the ability to bring to one's doorstep the 'face of the HIV/AIDS epidemic' while providing people living with HIV the comfort of visual anonymity."

The start-up process for the radio serial involved meeting with representatives from All India Radio and selecting people living with HIV to serve as radio journalists. The latter group participated in a three-day training on equipment use, interviewing techniques, and communication skills. During that time, TCH and NMP+ conducted a workshop to identify priority themes and issues to be covered in the serial. They then produced a design document outlining key content and messages, which served as an essential reference guide in the field for the radio journalists and the scriptwriter.

The team developed and tested the initial four episodes for audience feedback and used their input to inform the development of the remaining episodes. Key insights from audience testing included the following:

- The desire of the audience to hear more about the HIV-positive person's story, in addition to that of the person who supported him or her.
- The importance of stating up front that the interviewer is living with HIV, which helps dispel the misconception that people living with HIV are sick and unable to contribute to society. One respondent said, "I get gooseflesh on hearing that the person doing the interview is herself [HIV] positive. . . . [T]his is something that's quite unbelievable . . . how you overcome your own problem and then take part in this program."
- A need to provide more in-depth information on HIV transmission, prevention, and treatment. For example, one respondent wondered

how Sandeep, who learned he had HIV at age 12, could be infected since he had not been sexually active.

- A need to include information on where the audience could seek testing and treatment and on how to locate the nearest branch of NMP+.
- The need to help journalists improve the sound quality of their interviews.

Results

Radio journalists, people interviewed by the radio journalists, and TCH team members all talked about their own learning and growth through participation in this project.

People living with HIV who were trained to be radio journalists discussed the technical skills they learned (for example, use of computers and digital recorders). One explained, "I was not acquainted to a computer before [but] learned from this project because I had to download and send the files to Mumbai."

They also learned interviewing techniques: "I learned how to concentrate doing the interviews. Listening is an art, if you are doing an interview—you need to listen." They gained skills in public speaking, articulating questions, and delivering messages. One radio journalist who conducted the studio interviews with invited experts emphasized how great it made her feel to be the one doing the interviewing for a change:

> I have always been the interviewed, not the person doing the interviews. I learned how to interview. Now I understand all these technical things—for example, differences between conducting interviews in the field and in the studio. I feel really great [said with a huge smile] about being in the position to ask the questions, since I am always answering questions. But I also learned a lot about how difficult it is to do good interviews, that there [are] lots of skills needed.

Those interviewed often found the process powerful and rewarding. The radio journalists felt the interviews were often cathartic. The journalists found that interviewees were proud that their story was important enough to be on radio and were pleased that others would benefit from hearing it. As one radio journalist explained:

> I interviewed Sakshi's brother-in-law and mother-in-law. They said that if this message can go to the society and others can start caring for their positive family member that would make them feel good. It was also a good experience

for Sakshi and her mother-in-law. . . . [B]efore the interview she was taking care of Sakshi but not talking about [Sakshi's HIV-positive status] openly. So the interview helped to open up a channel of communication. It definitely improved [the] relationship between daughter-in-law and mother-in-law.

This story is particularly powerful because it highlights a scenario that goes against the norm: most in-laws tend to reject a daughter-in-law living with HIV.

An HIV counselor working with children who was interviewed for one of the studio episodes noted that the interview provided an opportunity for her to sharpen her advocacy skills:

This was the first time I've been for a recording like this. I enjoyed it. It made me speak clearly, learn how to pass on the message better. It provided me with confidence and skills to do other interviews and get across my message more effectively.

For TCH project team members, the project has been a learning process, not only about HIV, but also about the damaging impacts of stigma and discrimination and the benefits of care and support. As the producer of the radio series stated:

I learned a lot about HIV. I knew basic things, like not spreading by touch. But in-depth things—about society and the people and how they react—I didn't know these things. Knowing that you have this kind of support available [networks] is a big thing. I didn't know that so many organizations were out there to help [HIV-positive] people.

Team members also gained newfound respect for the strength of the people they met living with HIV. The scriptwriter explained:

They have given me so much, these stories. Many of the people being interviewed come from disadvantaged or less privileged groups, and against all odds, with their [HIV-positive] status and society having such negative attitudes, . . . they have taken their life in hand and are moving forward. It is quite inspiring.

Lessons Learned

Team members learned several key lessons during the development of the radio serial that can inform similar projects in the future.

Training and Support Need to Be Ongoing

Although the radio journalists greatly appreciated the initial three-day training, all agreed that if they had the opportunity to do it over, the training would be much longer. They also recommended mentoring on recording techniques (such as how to minimize ambient noise) and interviewing techniques (such as how to ask shorter and sharper questions). They also felt that refresher training would be useful after a few initial interviews. Specific suggestions included longer training with more practice sessions, more training on the equipment, and studio visits to understand the issues surrounding background noise and sound disturbances.

Care Should Be Taken to Ensure That Stigmatizing Language Is Not Used

As part of the training workshop, the full team had a brainstorming session on harmful words that are frequently used in the media and daily discourse and tried to find better alternatives. They then devised guidelines to ensure that stigmatizing language would not be used in interviews. As one radio journalist explained:

> As [HIV-positive] persons, we are always pointing out to the media the issues with their coverage, how it stigmatizes us, the words they use. So with this project, we have taken very great care in words we use so we lead by example. [We] show what other words that are not stigmatizing can be used—that it is possible to still communicate effectively without using stigmatizing words.

Many People Are Still Reluctant to Be Interviewed or Portrayed

Strong role models (that is, those who supported people living with HIV) were often reluctant to be interviewed for fear of what might happen when the story was broadcast:

> When we were first told to get 13 to 15 stories, we thought it would be easy, but it was actually very difficult because getting consent from the role models was hard. . . . People are ready to support the person living with HIV privately, but to do it publicly is not so easy. They fear experiencing stigma and discrimination.

More broadly, the project team found that one theme they could not cover was the workplace setting. Employers were reluctant to discuss programs and policies for staff members living with HIV, because they felt it would send a message that they employed many HIV-positive people, which they feared might hurt their corporate image and product sales.

To respond to this challenge and also to ensure that the project responded to the identified need for more factual information on HIV (for example, information about counseling and testing, mother-to-child transmission of HIV, and HIV treatment), the project team arranged a few studio interviews with experts to cover those topics.

Benefits of and Strategies for a Successful Partnership

Central to the success of project implementation has been the partnership between TCH and NMP+. Representatives of both organizations described the importance of this partnership and the benefits, learning, and inspiration it brought. The NMP+ project coordinator emphasized that once the radio serial aired, it would bring increased visibility to NMP+. Not only would the serial inform people living with HIV and their families about the network, but it would also encourage other agencies to partner with NMP+.

The project also strengthened participants' understanding of how to forge a productive partnership. The memorandum of understanding (MOU) signed at the start of the project was key to the partnership's success. It was jointly created by the two organizations, thereby ensuring equal buy-in up front, and it clearly laid out expectations, roles, and responsibilities. The NMP+ project coordinator explained, "The MOU was an important piece that we made together, as mutual understanding should be there. It should not happen that an organization should create [an] MOU and the network just signs." The working relationship also emphasized ongoing communication, joint decision making, and mutual respect.

Recommendations

Although TCH and NMP+ representatives said that their partnership would endure beyond the project and that they hoped others would replicate the project, they also noted ways in which it could be improved. Their recommendations include being more realistic about the timeline, logistics, and budget. Specifically, they pointed to the need to select sites that were closer together to allow hands-on field support. They also suggested building in more time both to account for possible delays resulting from consent refusal or health issues and to provide more in-depth training. Finally, they suggested ensuring the budget was sufficient to cover the broadcasting and evaluation of the radio serial.

CHAPTER 11

Ensuring Dignity and Rights among Female Sex Workers in Bangalore: A Community-Led Advocacy Campaign to Reduce Stigma and Discrimination

Women sex workers living with HIV face multiple stigmas that prevent them from sharing their status and accessing needed care, even within a supportive environment. For many women, the stigma can mean an untimely and unnecessary death. Such was the case for Revamma, a 29-year-old woman who turned to sex work when faced with the challenge of raising her children alone after her husband abandoned her. In her spare time, she volunteered as a peer educator to inform other women in sex work about HIV and AIDS—so her death from complications caused by HIV infection was a shock to her peers. Apparently, the fear of experiencing even more stigma and discrimination than she already faced as a sex worker led her to conceal her HIV status.

Revamma's story was the inspiration for Project Baduku, an effort funded by the South Asia Region Development Marketplace (SARDM) that aimed to empower and build the capacity of women in sex work to challenge stigma and discrimination. Project Baduku led advocacy efforts directed toward the general public and secondary stakeholders, such as police and health care workers, and toward the partners, family members, and neighbors of women in sex work. The campaigns sought to sensitize these populations about the issues women in sex work and people living with HIV face and to encourage change in societal attitudes and biases. As part of this process, the project aimed to provide opportunities for (a) interaction between the sex worker community and stakeholders in a noncontextual scenario (for example, outside of hospitals and police stations); (b) intercommunity dialogue and discussions among women in sex work about experiences of stigma and discrimination; and (c) capacity strengthening and leadership development in the sex worker community to strengthen processes related to decision making, management, implementation, and self-governance. The project was envisioned and implemented by three support organizations for women in sex work in urban Bangalore—Swathi Mahila Sangha, Vijaya Mahila Sangha, and Jyothi Mahila Sangha—with technical support from the Swasti Health Resource Center, a local nongovernmental organization (NGO).

Implementation

The project began with formative research to inform the content of advocacy messages and determine the target populations. The level and main sources of stigma and discrimination among women in sex work were assessed using data collected from 166 women in sex work at drop-in centers. Data were collected through an innovative pictorial questionnaire appropriate for female sex workers with minimal literacy skills. Responses to this questionnaire highlighted the need to address internalized stigma among women in sex work and sex workers living with HIV. In addition, the data identified key secondary stakeholders to target for advocacy.

The next step was to recruit and train the project staff, which included 15 community mobilizers and a project coordinator from the three implementing partners' support organizations. All were women in sex work, and most were living with HIV. The women were provided with leadership training and training on stigma and discrimination. Project staff members then led advocacy events, approached secondary stakeholders (police and health workers) to discourage stigma, and worked with families and neighbors of women in sex work to address reported cases of stigma and discrimination. In addition, project staff members supported and worked to strengthen the capacity of women sex workers living with HIV. They helped train more than 400 staff members from the project's three implementing support organizations on stigma and discrimination so the latter could participate in the various advocacy events held around Bangalore.

All the advocacy campaigns were designed to highlight the positive role the public and secondary stakeholders can play in improving the lives of women in sex work, rather than blaming such stakeholders for stigma and discrimination. The project reached out to the public through campaigns such as the Signature campaign, the Human Chain campaign, and the Handshake campaign. By facilitating contact between the public and women in sex work living with HIV, these campaigns helped address fears and misconceptions about HIV transmission and vulnerable groups. Other campaigns targeted specific stakeholders. In the Bike campaign, for example, hundreds of women in sex work and supporters of the stigma reduction efforts biked to hospitals around the city to engage medical professionals in discussing the issues facing women sex workers living with HIV. The Rose campaign recognized doctors and police who had been particularly supportive and sensitive to the sex worker community and requested their help in convincing their colleagues to be similarly supportive. Project staff members also presented roses to some people who had been particularly stigmatizing and abusive in the past to encourage behavior change among these individuals.

In addition to these advocacy campaigns, project staff members engaged in targeted advocacy as needed. For example, community mobilizers responded to specific cases of discrimination reported by female sex workers, such as isolation by family members and avoidance by neighbors. The crisis response teams were also trained to identify and respond to cases of discrimination. Last, the project continuously reached out to the media to expand the reach of advocacy messages, for example, by informing the media about the location and times of all public advocacy events to enhance press coverage. In addition, the project partnered with the Centre for Advocacy and Research to prepare several of the project staff members living with HIV for specific media events, including television, radio, and newspaper interviews and press conferences.

Results

Overall, the project was quite successful. More than 220 campaigns were conducted throughout Bangalore reaching more than 2,150 secondary stakeholders. During the Signature campaign, 132,000 individuals signed their name and pledged not to stigmatize or discriminate against women in sex work, and more than 225,000 individuals were reached in the other campaigns. The project's simple and quick advocacy approaches inspired cooperation and support and helped change negative attitudes and behaviors among the public and secondary stakeholders. The project's advocacy efforts also boosted confidence among sex workers living with HIV, who were not used to receiving such support and encouragement. Expressing how participating in the project changed her life, one of the community mobilizers living with HIV said:

> Being a part of Project Baduku gave me the mental stamina I needed to resist stigma and discrimination and deal with my disease. It made me strong. When you are better mentally, you are better physically.

The Rose campaign was particularly effective at reaching secondary stakeholders. Evidence suggests that following the campaign, sex workers were more comfortable reporting cases of stigma and discrimination, because the number of cases they reported to the police grew from 0 to 11. Furthermore, the police actively responded to and resolved all of these cases, a strong testament to their willingness to take complaints from sex workers seriously. In addition, sex workers anecdotally reported less harassment and violence from police following the advocacy campaign in a jurisdiction where violence had previously been quite high.

In the health care setting, the percentage of HIV-positive female sex workers from the three support organizations who regularly sought care and treatment services at antiretroviral therapy centers in Bangalore increased from 30 percent before the project to 60 percent during and after. Women appeared to be more comfortable sharing their HIV status with their families and the project staff. Overall, health care workers responded positively to the campaign. The head of the antiretroviral therapy department at Kempegowda Institute of Medical Sciences Hospital in Bangalore said that members of the medical staff were motivated to see such dedication from the sex worker community and that this dedication has inspired them to advocate on their behalf. "Since the campaign, we began advising women to go to the Lawyer's Collective to seek help for violence issues," he said. "We are also sending students for training at Swathi Mahila Sangha to better understand the issues facing women in sex work."

The campaigns also provided accurate information about how HIV is and is not transmitted, which quelled the fears of members of the public, such as this taxi driver, who attended a sensitization meeting held near his taxi stand:

> Many auto drivers do not know how HIV spreads. They think that it is contagious by touching those with HIV. After Project Baduku, at least 10 to 15 auto drivers in this area are more sensitive to HIV-positive women in sex work. We have taken patients [with HIV] to the hospital for checkup just like any other patients. Earlier, probably many of us would refuse. In addition, many of us have got [our] blood tested for HIV.

As a result of the strategic media engagement, more than 20 articles were published in both local-language and English-language newspapers, and a local television station aired a program developed by Swathi Mahila Sangha called *Jagruthi* (*Seven Days*) about HIV and women in sex work. In addition, one of the community mobilizers participated in a televised interview, another participated in a radio interview, and seven project staff members participated in two live press conferences.

Lessons Learned

One of the key lessons learned was the value of mobilizing the community affected by stigma and discrimination to lead a movement against this problem. Before Project Baduku, three support organizations for women in sex work were working separately in different areas of Bangalore. Because of their collective recognition of the need to foster a more supportive environment for women in sex work, these organizations joined together, with support from the NGO Swasti, to write the SARDM proposal. The resulting partnership among the four organizations proved critical for implementing and monitoring a large and multifaceted campaign. Project Baduku staff members were immediately able to train the existing staff from the three support organizations, which enabled quick scale-up of the intervention and ensured that the advocacy messages reached all corners of the city. This effort helped maximize the benefits of stigma reduction for the 24,000 women in sex work in the city. As a direct result of this project, the three support organizations have launched the Network for Women's Equity and Equality, which they hope will become a regional or national umbrella organization for sex worker support organizations throughout the country. The success of this partnership demonstrates the value in fostering partnerships between community-based organizations and technical NGOs for the design and implementation of stigma reduction efforts.

Strengthening the capacity of women in sex work living with HIV to lead stigma reduction efforts proved both motivating and inspiring. Many of the women reported newfound confidence and courage, which enabled them to confront stigma and discrimination in their own lives and to become advocates for the rights of others. The commitment of the HIV-positive women leading the project to proactively engage with stakeholders and try to improve their environment motivated many stakeholders to join the women in support of their stigma reduction efforts.

The success of the advocacy campaigns also can be attributed to the regular staff training, which ensured staff members' mastery of basic themes and issues pertaining to HIV and sex worker stigma. Such knowledge was needed to execute the campaigns effectively. Regular steering committee meetings were also important to review results and adapt advocacy campaigns and messages as needed. For example, engaging health care providers and police in the large public campaigns was very challenging. Therefore, project staff members decided to craft a more personalized one-to-one campaign to ensure that they could reach these groups, which have particular influence over the treatment and well-being of sex workers.

A strategy for engaging with the media was also crucial. To ensure press coverage of the advocacy campaigns, project staff members informed the media prior to the events and regularly updated them on the campaign outcomes. In addition, project staff members were well prepared to engage the media in interviews and public forums. These efforts ensured that the issue of HIV-related stigma and discrimination received wider publicity and visibility and strengthened the capacity of women in sex work to speak out openly and advocate for their rights. Last, a key lesson learned was that addressing morality-related stigma and discrimination requires multiple approaches and takes time. Thus, maintaining stigma reduction efforts in the longer term and adapting advocacy strategies to match the key concerns of specific target audiences are critical.

PART III

Project Summaries of the 26 Stigma Reduction Projects

CHAPTER 12

Afghanistan

Afghan Family Guidance Association

Project title: HIV and AIDS Stigma and Discrimination Reduction through Raising Awareness in Kabul City, Afghanistan

Implementing organization: Afghan Family Guidance Association (AFGA)

Location: Kabul

Background

Program goals: To address two prevailing root causes of HIV-related stigma and discrimination in Afghan society: (a) lack of accurate knowledge and information on HIV and (b) misconceptions regarding Islamic principles and cultural beliefs

Target audiences: Health workers, youth, prisoners, prison staff members (medical and nonmedical), religious leaders, and media representatives

Primary approaches: Training and knowledge sharing

Description of intervention: AFGA conducted several trainings on HIV stigma reduction with various target groups, including AFGA service providers, youth peer educators, medical and nonmedical prison staff members, peer educators in prison, religious leaders, and members of the media. The project compiled training materials from the Web site of the Joint United Nations Programme on HIV/AIDS and other sources and translated these items into the local language. Two-day trainings on HIV and AIDS and stigma reduction were conducted with 60 AFGA service providers and 25 members of the medical staff of prison health centers. The project also conducted one-day trainings with 91 nonmedical prison staff members, 28 prisoner peer educators, and 13 AFGA youth peer educators. Initially, the team trained 25 religious leaders from the Ministry of Haj and Religious Affairs. The project team then decided that rolling out the training would be more effective if it were led by senior religious leaders, so AFGA trained three additional senior religious leaders from the Ministry of Haj and Religious Affairs responsible for mosque-related issues. These senior religious leaders then trained 75 junior religious leaders throughout Kabul with technical support from AFGA. In all, the project trained 103 religious leaders. AFGA also produced a television (TV) spot on HIV, AIDS, and stigma that the media broadcast widely.

Recognizing the powerful role of religious leaders in influencing the public in Afghan society, the project initiated collaboration with senior religious leaders from the Ministry of Haj and Religious Affairs. The project increased awareness among religious leaders about HIV, AIDS, and stigma and provided guidance on disseminating such messages to the public through Friday prayer (*khutba*). Training materials were developed that included guidance for religious leaders on the importance of health as one of the gifts from Allah and the four common transmission routes of HIV. In addition, the training materials included three *hadiths* that encourage Muslims to show sympathy for ill people and to help those people in any way they can. The overall objective was to convey the message that AIDS is a disease like other diseases and that people living with HIV and AIDS should be accorded behavior that avoids stigma and discrimination. The materials were approved by the National AIDS Control Program Directorate of the Ministry of Public Health of Afghanistan and formally sent by the General Directorate of Mosques of the Ministry of Haj and Religious Affairs to mosques in Kabul for use as material for Friday prayer talks. The materials are currently available in Dari. TV channels were then informed of the dates for Friday prayers containing HIV awareness messages and were requested to record and broadcast the talks so a wider audience could be reached. At least three TV channels, including the national TV channel, broadcast the talks.

The project also took initial steps to establish a partnership with the media. Sixty media representatives participated in a two-day sensitization training, and journalists were encouraged to start broadcasting stigma reduction messages, including the TV spot that was developed through the project.

In addition to the trainings, the project developed information, education, and communication (IEC) and behavior change communication (BCC) materials (in collaboration with the Ministry of Public Health), including leaflets, two posters, and a TV spot. Peer educators helped distribute the IEC and BCC materials.

Implementation, Results, and Challenges

Measurement strategies: Pre- and posttraining evaluation assessments were conducted with 40 AFGA service providers (doctors, midwives, and counselors); 18 prison medical staff members; 13 AFGA peer educators; and 58 journalists. The survey included 20 true/false questions, and scores were generated on the basis of the responses. Higher scores reflected better knowledge of HIV and AIDS and greater awareness and understanding of stigma and discrimination.

AFGA conducted four focus group discussions with specific target groups: prison staff members, health service providers, peer educators (prisoners), and youth peer educators. Information was gathered on (a) general knowledge of HIV and AIDS, prevention, and modes of transmission; (b) stigma and discrimination toward people living with HIV and AIDS; (c) availability of IEC materials; and (d) roles of health service providers in reducing stigma and discrimination. In addition, the facilitators encouraged focus group participants to provide information on common challenges in reducing stigma and discrimination in Afghan society and their recommendations for improving current efforts.

Results, key findings, and lessons: In all, 320 key stakeholders participated in training events held throughout the project. On average, the training evaluations demonstrated an increase in knowledge of HIV and AIDS and awareness of stigma and discrimination. Analysis of the focus group discussions revealed that most of the target groups had basic awareness of information regarding HIV and AIDS and stigma and discrimination. The analysis suggested that ignorance, low awareness, and misconceptions were the main sources of stigma and discrimination toward people living with HIV and AIDS. The analysis also suggested that comprehensive awareness-raising programs using culturally appropriate IEC and BCC materials and involvement of religious leaders (disseminating messages through mosques) and the media were effective approaches to address these sensitive issues. One example of the improved attitudes among trained stakeholders involved a female prisoner living with HIV who was on antiretroviral treatment. A prison medical staff member explained how when the patient needed intravenous (IV) rehydration, nobody from the female prison health staff was comfortable putting in an IV line. After discussion with the project staff, the prison medical staff agreed to provide the IV therapy. Since receiving the training, health staff members regularly visit this patient without showing any discriminatory behavior.

AFGA received positive feedback from audience members on the TV spot it prepared and broadcast on stigma. Those giving favorable comments included the Ministry of Public Health and other stakeholders working on HIV and AIDS. It is the first time such a TV spot has been broadcast in Afghanistan, especially on stigma. The feedback noted the clarity of the contents and its suitability in the Afghanistan context.

Challenges and unforeseen outcomes: Challenges included security restrictions and lengthy administrative procedures to get authorities to approve project members' working in a prison setting. To address this issue, AFGA held consecutive coordination meetings with prison authorities and provided detailed information on the goals and objectives of the project and the benefits for the prisoners and the prison staff. Prison authorities were involved in each step of project implementation.

Encouraging the involvement of religious leaders in the trainings was also challenging at times. Awareness of HIV and stigma was generally low among the mullahs. Most linked HIV with sexual behaviors that are not acceptable by Sharia (Islamic) law. The project team used a number of strategies to encourage participation, including showing gentle persistence; meeting religious leaders on their own ground (for example, using Islamic holy texts to illustrate why religious leaders should consider the project's message and engage with the project team); appealing to the compassionate side that exists in all religions; and asking for help in a nonthreatening and nonjudgmental way. The collaborative relationship between AFGA and the Ministry of Haj and Religious Affairs helped facilitate involvement of religious leaders in the trainings.

Additional Information
Program references, media coverage, and materials developed:

- *How to Behave towards People Living with HIV and AIDS from the Islamic Perspective* (training materials in Dari)
- Dari translation of *Understanding and Challenging HIV Stigma Toolkit,* module 3, chapter A, "HIV Stigma—Naming and Owning the Problem," and module 4, chapter B, "Gender Violence—Naming and Owning the Problem"
- Report on findings from focus group discussions

Contact information: Naimatullah Akbari, nakbari@afga.org.af

Additional funding, replication, or scale-up opportunities or new partnerships resulting from the project: AFGA is currently partnering with Futures Group International to implement a mass media campaign using print, radio, and TV to broadcast HIV and AIDS–related messages to the general public. Thus far, two individuals from each type of media have been trained as focal persons on health issues—and HIV and AIDS in particular. In addition, AFGA has received one year of additional funding from the Afghanistan office of the United Nations Office on Drugs and Crime (UNODC) to continue working in the women's prison of Kabul on HIV and AIDS–related issues.

Afghan Help and Training Program

Project title: Tackling HIV and AIDS Stigma and Discrimination: From Insight to Action

Implementing organization: Afghan Help and Training Program (AHTP)

Location: Jalalabad, Nangarhar province

Background
Program goals: To raise awareness of stigma and discrimination in the context of HIV and AIDS

Target audiences: Religious leaders, mullahs and mawlawies, mosque congregations, and youth association leaders

Primary approaches: Training-of-trainers (TOT) and IEC materials

Description of intervention: AHTP designed a seven-day stigma and HIV and AIDS TOT curriculum, which consisted of modules on (a) general information about HIV, AIDS, sexually transmitted infections, and tuberculosis; (b) attitudes toward people living with HIV; (c) stigma and discrimination in Islam; (d) HIV and AIDS in Islam; and (e) the role of religious leaders in combating HIV and AIDS. Training modules included specific texts from the Koran to support the reduction of stigma. Experts from the government, such as representatives of the provincial offices of the Ministry of Public Health and the Ministry of Haj and Religious Affairs and the National AIDS Control Program (NACP), as well as experts from local universities in Nangarhar, reviewed and approved the modules.

When the training materials were approved, the project trained 10 senior and well-respected religious leaders as master trainers. Officially, 300 mullahs and mawlawies (senior to mullahs in knowledge) are assigned by the government to the city of Jalalabad, yet the city has many other mullahs, including those in seminaries. The master trainers, with support from the project team, trained all 300 officially assigned mullahs and mawlawies in Jalalabad under the strict supervision and monitoring of the NACP. In addition to providing the trainings, the project organized large gatherings led by the master trainers in which mullahs and mawlawies, some of whom had participated in the training and others who were invited from neighboring districts, were sensitized about HIV and the related stigma and discrimination. These gatherings reached approximately 400 mullahs and mawlawies throughout Jalalabad. Attendees agreed to fight against HIV and AIDS–related stigma and discrimination.

The project held monthly coordination meetings with key stakeholders to share experiences and improve project implementation. These stakeholders included representatives from the provincial public health directorate and HIV and AIDS implementing partners in the province such as the United Nations Children's Fund (UNICEF), BRAC, HealthNet International and the Transcultural Psycho-social Organisation (HNI-TPO), and the Swedish Committee. Although the project team did not initially include youth associations as targets for trainings, these groups were added because senior religious leaders recommended them as an important audience to reach with antistigma messages. A three-day training led by AHTP was conducted for top-level members of youth associations (including males and females) throughout Jalalabad to increase knowledge and awareness of HIV and AIDS and stigma and to enhance HIV prevention among youth.

Implementation, Results, and Challenges

Measurement strategies: Pre- and posttraining evaluations were conducted among the 300 mullahs and mawlawies who participated in the training. The highest achievable score was 100, reflecting correct responses to all of the knowledge and awareness questions. At pretest, 19 percent of participants provided correct responses, compared with 72 percent at posttest, with an average increase of 53 percentage points following the training. Preintervention (baseline) and postintervention (end-line) surveys were also conducted.

Results, key findings, and lessons: The project successfully secured the commitment of the government, mullahs, and local communities to reduce HIV stigma and discrimination. A strong coordinating body for the project was effectively developed and 18 monthly coordination meetings were held. The project effectively involved government and community authorities in project planning, implementation, and decision making. The trained mullahs effectively conveyed messages to community members, and community awareness of HIV- and stigma-related issues increased as a result. The project conveyed messages on HIV, AIDS, and stigma to more than 45,000 people in five districts of Jalalabad and distributed 5,000 posters and 60,000 leaflets. The messages were designed to allay fears about HIV transmission through casual contact with a person living with HIV and called for compassionate treatment of HIV-positive people. The project conveyed these messages with support from texts in the Koran and speeches of Prophet Muhammad.

Challenges and unforeseen outcomes: Specific challenges mentioned by project staff members included a low level of knowledge about HIV and AIDS and stigma and discrimination among religious leaders. HIV is strongly linked to sexual practices that are illegal in Afghanistan, and other modes of transmission are not well known. Many religious leaders expressed concern that participating in the training would result in their being isolated by their community for raising the issues of HIV and stigma or would cause them to lose their jobs. To overcome this obstacle, AHTP held several coordinating meetings with religious leaders in the provincial offices of the Ministry of Haj and Religious Affairs, where they held long discussions about HIV, AIDS, and stigma. Once these leaders were convinced of the importance of conveying this information, the project sought official approval from the Ministry of Haj and Religious Affairs in Kabul for the training activities. The ministry in Kabul reassured training participants through a written agreement, which contained approval from both the ministry in Kabul and the provincial offices, that the training materials reflected the teachings of the Koran and that it was the responsibility of religious leaders to help prevent the spread of HIV by conveying the messages learned in the training. After the TOT program was under way, the training participants became more confident and gained more knowledge about HIV and AIDS. They requested additional reference materials on HIV and AIDS and stigma in particular. They even developed a strategy for reducing stigma and increasing knowledge of HIV and AIDS. Some trainers were invited to appear on local radio and TV shows with the support of local government.

Another challenge arose during the review of training materials by government and religious officials. The officials expressed some initial concern over the stigma reduction modules specifically, so the project team decided to increase the knowledge of religious leaders about HIV and AIDS first and then teach them about HIV-related stigma and discrimination.

Additional Information

Program references, media coverage, and materials developed:

- TOT package for senior religious leaders
- Training package for religious leaders
- *Understanding and Challenging Stigma Toolkit*, shared with the NACP and then translated and distributed to the 10 trainers
- IEC materials consisting of leaflets and posters

Contact information: Amanullah Momand, dramanullah_momand@ yahoo.com

Additional funding, replication, or scale-up opportunities or new partnerships resulting from the project: The NACP supports replicating the TOT strategy and project activities in other parts of the country. Accordingly, AHTP plans to replicate this intervention in five more districts of Nangarhar province, as well as in other provinces of the country.

A number of important partnerships have also arisen as a result of the intervention, including a partnership between the NACP and the Ministry of Haj and Religious Affairs. In addition, a partnership of community leaders has been established. By working with the communities of the districts in Nangarhar province, AHTP has established relationships, close contacts, and cooperation with elders of these communities and has established a good reputation in the region, which will enable expansion of the project into other areas.

Concern Worldwide

Project title: Addressing HIV and AIDS Related Stigma and Discrimination in Afghanistan

Implementing organizations: Concern Worldwide, ActionAid Afghanistan, Just Afghan Capacity and Knowledge (JACK)

Location: Kabul, Takhar, Badakshan, Nangarhar, Konar, Balkh, and Herat provinces

Background

Program goals: To address stigma and discrimination associated with HIV and AIDS in Afghanistan, to facilitate training of key groups and individuals to reduce stigma and discrimination, and to support the formation of a network of people living with HIV in Afghanistan

Target audiences: Health professionals, mullahs, teachers, prison officers, community leaders, police officers, and people living with HIV

Primary approaches: Film and training

Description of intervention: The project supported the development and production of six research and training films on stigma and HIV and AIDS. The research and training films were informed by formative research among individuals living with HIV and AIDS. In addition, film scripts were developed through extensive consultation among project staff members, researchers, and the media company. The films, produced in two local languages (Pashto and Dari), are the first of their kind in Afghanistan to deal with HIV-related stigma and discrimination. The films were tested among six groups before completion. These groups included mullahs, teachers, prison and police officers, community leaders, and health professionals, across districts and urban centers including Kabul and Herat. The films were then incorporated into a training course on HIV and AIDS. In addition to producing the films and conducting trainings, the project commissioned an artist to develop posters and leaflets with messages promoting awareness of HIV-related stigma.

Implementation, Results, and Challenges

Measurement strategies: Formative research was conducted with 27 people living with HIV using a structured questionnaire. Themes covered in the questionnaire included individuals' experiences of stigma and discrimination as well as their interest in forming a group for individuals living with HIV and AIDS. The results of this survey informed the development of the films.

To measure the effectiveness of the training course, project staff members administered a questionnaire that assessed the knowledge of the participants in each of the groups before and after showing the research films and training the participants on HIV and AIDS.

Results, key findings, and lessons: During the course of the project, 354 individuals from six groups viewed the films and received training on HIV and AIDS. This process was facilitated by the ministries, including the Ministry of Haj and Religious Affairs. In addition, the films were field-tested with additional groups of religious leaders—40 in Kabul and 43 in the northern province of Takhar—and were shown to a group of TV, radio, and print media personnel.

The films were universally well received by all the groups and were thought to be sensitively made and culturally and religiously appropriate, especially by the mullahs. The films showing family dynamics, such as those between an HIV-positive wife and an HIV-positive husband, produced a very sympathetic reaction in the audiences. The comedy films, which made fun of prejudiced village leaders, greatly amused all the groups.

Pre- and posttest results: All trainees were assessed at the start and at the end of the course. Table 12.1 and figure 12.1 show the results of these assessments. A total of 245 trainees satisfactorily completed the pre- and posttests. A further 109 were trained but were not able to participate in the pre- and posttesting either because they were illiterate or because they answered the questionnaires incompletely (see table 12.1). Figure 12.1 represents those who completed the questionnaires.

Table 12.1   Trainee Groups

Trainee group	People who completed pre- and posttest training	Additional people trained but who could not satisfactorily complete the test
Community leaders	29	18
Health professionals	47	0
Police officers	21	23
Prison officers	26	23
Religious leaders	99	34
Teachers	23	11
Total	245	109

Sources: Concern Worldwide and Action Aid, Afghanistan.

Figure 12.1   Pre- and Postcourse Assessment Results

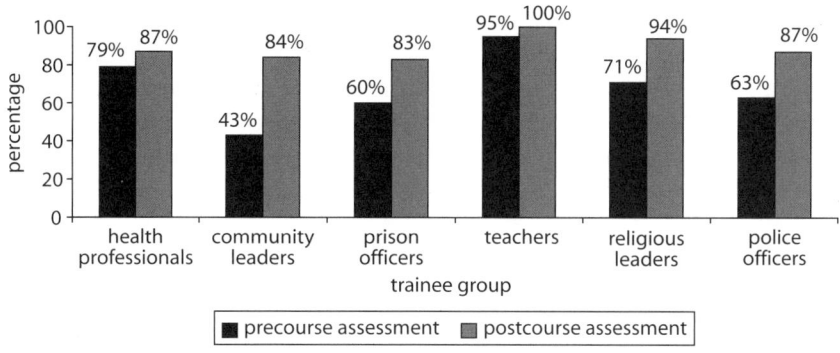

Sources: Concern Worldwide and Action Aid, Afghanistan.

The results of the project and the films were presented to an audience of nongovernmental organization representatives, officials of the Ministry of Public Health, and members of various United Nations organizations. On the basis of the request of the majority of the HIV-positive people interviewed during the project, a group for people living with HIV was established. The formation of the first network of individuals living with HIV and AIDS in Afghanistan was an important outcome of the project. The work accomplished through the Ministry of Haj and Religious Affairs to enable the films to be shown to religious leaders was also important.

Challenges and unforeseen outcomes: The main challenges faced during the project included locating and interviewing individuals living with HIV and AIDS. Participants were recruited through voluntary counseling and testing centers. A majority of the HIV-positive individuals included in the research were injecting drug users, reflecting the epidemiological pattern of infection in Afghanistan. Injecting drug users are already stigmatized in Afghanistan, and HIV compounds the stigma experienced by this group. Researchers purposely tried to recruit HIV-positive participants who were not injecting drug users. The original number of researchers involved in the project was reduced from four to two because of the difficulty in identifying researchers with the appropriate skills and background.

Additional Information

Program references, media coverage, and materials developed: Six films in Pashto and Dari

Contact information: Fiona McLysaght, Fiona.McLysaght@concern.net

Additional funding, replication, or scale-up opportunities or new partnerships resulting from the project: Concern Worldwide is seeking additional funding for the reproduction and dissemination of the training course films from UNICEF and UNODC in Kabul. Concern Worldwide intends to show the films on national TV and adapt them for radio. They will also be used by the NACP and nongovernmental organizations working in the field.

CHAPTER 13

Bangladesh

Drik Picture Library

Project title: Mainstreaming the Fringe

Implementing organization: Drik Picture Library

Location: Dhanmondi, Dhaka

Background

Program goal: To mainstream issues such as denial and stigma by expanding access to knowledge, so that sensitive topics related to HIV and AIDS are incorporated into everyday discourse. To accomplish this goal, Drik created a space and facilitated opportunities for the public, people with high visibility, disseminators, and educators, including journalists, filmmakers, and teachers, to engage on issues of vital concern that cannot typically be broadcast because of fear, vulnerability, and ignorance.

Target audiences: People with high visibility who may be seen as role models or activists; disseminators and educators, such as journalists, filmmakers, publishers, and teachers; and the general public

Primary approach: Media campaign

Description of intervention: The project developed a media campaign using traditional and new media, including Web-based and non-Web-based video and audio programs to raise awareness about HIV, AIDS, stigma, denial, and the challenges facing marginalized populations. The campaign included roundtable talk shows, oral testimonials, and news dissemination via the Web. This work involved setting up a recording studio. In addition, guidelines were developed for media messages related to HIV, AIDS, and stigma. These guidelines were based on the current guidelines of the Joint United Nations Programme on HIV/AIDS (UNAIDS) regarding appropriate HIV terminology and were disseminated to participating journalists.

The content of the programs focused mainly on issues of sexuality and access to information. Programs used experts—such as visual journalist Shahidul Alam; Dr. Nazrul Islam, Bangabandhu Sheikh Mujib Medical University; and Jeevani Fernando, manager of Drik's stigma reduction program—to communicate clear messages in nontechnical language to promote comprehension and understanding among lay audiences. The live nature of talk shows and other programming provided both active and passive communication, thereby allowing both anonymity and visibility during discussion and reflection on sensitive topics. The educational channel, Ujala TV (based in Dubai), broadcast productions of some of the programs throughout South Asia in local languages.

In consultation with media stakeholders, Drik identified key training needs for local journalists regarding techniques for interviewing, gathering information, and reporting on sensitive topics such as HIV and AIDS.

Implementation, Results, and Challenges

Measurement strategy: The activities were not evaluated.

Results, key findings, and lessons: The media campaign—"Mainstreaming the Fringe to Promote Stigma Reduction"—encouraged people from all walks of life to engage on issues related to HIV and AIDS that are of vital concern but that are sensitive topics and not easily discussed publicly. Online Webcasting commenced in January 2009, thereby increasing visibility and access to information related to HIV, AIDS, and stigma. However, the programs documenting the personal stories of people living with HIV have yet to be broadcast because of reluctance among the individuals featured to make themselves public in a Web domain that is accessible worldwide. This issue indicates that more work is needed to reduce stigma at the societal level and to strengthen the capacity of people living with HIV and marginalized populations to share their stories and advocate for their rights.

Challenges and unforeseen outcomes: Some of the challenges encountered by the project included developing rapport and trust among marginalized groups that experience stigma and discrimination. After Drik covered the 12th-year celebrations of Bandhu, the only gay society of Bangladesh, many more marginalized groups came to Drik to document their own stories, share challenges, and seek funds for their own initiatives. This exposure paved the way for Drik to reach hidden and underground groups that previously had no positive media outlook on their activities. However, although Drik was able to engage people living with HIV and marginalized populations to participate in interviews, none of the individuals who participated are thus far willing to have their stories broadcast online to an international audience. Drik is working closely with Bandhu to help people living with HIV come forward more openly. Given the more religiously conservative societal system in Bangladesh, this transformation may take some time.

Another challenge faced was the limited availability of new media dissemination equipment in Bangladesh and insufficient bandwidth for Webcasting. For example, initially Drik organized a workshop and test run of the online forum with its own online network, DrikNEWS, including an event management team, resource personnel from medical institutions, and journalists from the public. The challenge in engaging people from the marginalized communities was due to insufficient Internet bandwidth in localities and lack of information technology knowledge. These challenges were addressed by seeking better Internet providers and shopping for necessary equipment outside of Bangladesh.

During the course of the project, it became clear that journalists at all levels in Bangladesh needed specific training on techniques for conducting live interviews on video and in front of live audiences, engaging with vulnerable populations, reporting on sensitive topics such as HIV and AIDS, and using the latest electronic media technologies in their reporting. Hence, Drik and its educational wing, Pathshala, established a Media Academy in March 2010 to address the capacity-strengthening needs of local journalists. Thus far, the academy has brought in trainers from the Netherlands, the United Kingdom, and the United States to train local journalists on proper interviewing techniques and equipment use. The academy also provides training on appropriate media messaging when reporting on HIV, AIDS, and stigma in accordance with current

UNAIDS guidelines. Thus far, 20 journalists have been trained at the Media Academy.

It will be important, in future media campaigns such as this one, to assess the effect of Drik's approach to mainstreaming and providing space for dialogue on sensitive topics, such as stigma related to HIV and AIDS, by including monitoring and evaluation activities in the design.

Additional Information

Program references, media coverage, and materials developed:

- A documentary on the lives and activities of the gay society in Bangladesh, *Bandhu*, is in progress. Bandhu's 12th-year anniversary celebrations were exclusively documented by DrikTV.
- A DVD (digital video disc) on the life of the hijras, "Celebrating Womanhood," is available and can also be viewed on http://www.drik.tv.

Contact information: Jeevani Fernando, jeevani@drik.net

Additional funding, replication, or scale-up opportunities or new partnerships resulting from the project: The World Bank provided additional support to Drik to document the lessons learned from the South Asia Region Development Marketplace 2008 stigma reduction grants on video. Drik Audiovisuals has completed this work. The stories will be made available on http://www.drik.tv (currently the summary "Insight to Action" is available on this site).

Job Opportunity and Business Support–Bangladesh

Project title: Economic Rehabilitation of Intravenous Drug Users

Implementing organization: Job Opportunity and Business Support (JOBS) Bangladesh

Location: Dhaka

Background

Program goals: To provide former male injecting drug users (IDUs) with economic opportunities and facilitate their road to economic independence (a fundamental requirement for them to regain their self-esteem and dignity as productive members of society) and to facilitate their reconnection with family members, help them overcome internalized stigma, and raise awareness to fight HIV stigma and discrimination among the general public.

Target audiences: Male IDUs, store owners, and the general public

Primary approaches: Employment services, training, advocacy

Description of intervention: JOBS worked closely with rehabilitation centers in Dhaka to select former male IDUs for specialized job training coupled with a stigma reduction component. Of 52 former IDUs interviewed, 20 participants were selected on the basis of factors such as level of motivation, history of drug use, and history of violence. The JOBS staff then made arrangements with a mannequin company to hire former IDUs for factory work and begin a new production line. JOBS subsidized the former IDUs' salaries for the first three months of the project with the agreement that if workers achieved the technical skills and productivity expected by the end of the probation period, the firm would hire them. JOBS also assigned two dedicated staff members, who provided informal counseling to participants for the first six months and coordinated weekly visits from a rehabilitation center counselor.

Before working at the factory, participants completed a five-day course using the Workplace Discipline and Congenial Environment Curriculum. This training aimed to provide individuals with the requisite skills to be successful in a factory environment and a basic understanding of financial management to prepare them for their economic independence. A combination of didactic and participatory methods was used along with confidence-building exercises. Following the training, participants received hands-on instruction in the production of mannequins. Last, a focus group discussion was conducted to provide participants with information about HIV prevention and transmission and to dispel misconceptions.

As part of the project's stigma reduction component, the former IDUs produced 50 red mannequins to be used in advocacy efforts throughout Dhaka. In the second stage of the project, seven of the men who performed well during the first six months were selected for additional block-batik training to design clothes with red ribbons. These clothes were then displayed on the red mannequins developed by the former IDUs as part of an advocacy campaign. The project also conducted a mini-seminar to equip the training participants with accurate information regarding HIV and AIDS. Participants were encouraged to disseminate their knowledge and serve as role models and ambassadors and to start their own grassroots campaign to inspire other IDUs struggling to break the addiction cycle.

In the final stage of the project, JOBS organized an advocacy campaign in well-known stores throughout Dhaka, with strong support from boutique owners and local fashion designers, and from Bibi Russell, the United Nations ambassador for HIV and AIDS. At each store, a red mannequin wearing white clothes with red ribbon designs produced by the former IDUs was displayed alongside information on the project and on HIV, injecting drug use, and stigma and discrimination in Bangladesh. Information was provided in English and Bengali. JOBS provided store owners with basic information about HIV and the project so they could respond to customers' questions. Mannequins and advocacy materials were displayed at drug rehabilitation centers, social clubs, and hotels. They also were included in workshops for university students.

Implementation, Results, and Challenges
Measurement strategies:

- Baseline survey and key informant interviews to understand the issues former IDUs confront on a daily basis
- A focus group discussion with IDU participants to clarify and answer questions about HIV and AIDS

Results, key findings, and lessons: Twenty graduates from rehabilitation centers received job training. Of the 20 participants trained, two started their own business selling daily items, five moved to a job with a better salary, six shifted to another factory that opened up, and six were offered alternative job opportunities but opted to pursue their own interests and leads. Only one participant dropped out.

A total of 50 red mannequins for advocacy purposes were produced. The project also developed a sustainable production line in which profits from the sale of regular mannequins are reinvested to hire more former IDUs.

Seven former IDUs participated in the block-batik training and designed saris, t-shirts, and men's clothing with red ribbons to dress the mannequins. A mini-seminar to equip the training participants with accurate information regarding HIV and AIDS was also conducted, and participants were encouraged to disseminate their knowledge, to serve as role models and ambassadors, and to start their own grassroots campaign to inspire other

IDUs struggling to break the addiction cycle. The red mannequins were showcased in 26 locations for awareness and advocacy purposes and used in five presentations given at various locations around the city.

Of participants who were trained and employed through the program, 75 percent were accepted back into their families by the end of the project period. This acceptance occurred because the participants were able to regain trust by staying away from drugs and holding a steady job and were able to save money and contribute to the family income again. The fact that participants maintained employment and reintegrated into family life after the program ended indicates that negative attitudes about former drug users among employers and family members can shift with a combination of job training and confidence-building interventions for former IDUs.

Job training combined with confidence-building efforts also helped participants overcome the internal stigma that kept them from succeeding in the past, and it enabled them to demonstrate that they can be productive members of society again.

Challenges and unforeseen outcomes: Although the red mannequins succeeded at attracting attention, how effective this strategy was at changing negative attitudes toward former IDUs is unclear. Mainly high-end shops participated in the advocacy campaign. Shop owners noted that few people asked questions about the project or the information presented. Former IDUs suggested that in the future the campaign should be expanded to include shops catering to a wider spectrum of society. In addition, the former IDUs would appreciate the opportunity to be more involved in advocacy and outreach efforts.

Finally, the sustainability of job skills and employment support projects for IDUs is clearly a challenge. At the start of the project, the private sector partner that was initially identified was reluctant to commit to investing in and starting a new production unit, so JOBS had to identify a new option. However, the partner company sold the mannequin production unit after the project ended, which resulted in job loss for several participants.

Additional Information

Program references, media coverage, and materials developed:

- Magazine article
- Final evaluation report

Contact information: Elli Takagaki, elli@jobs-ict.com; info@jobs-group.org

Additional funding, replication, or scale-up opportunities or new partnerships resulting from the project: JOBS-Bangladesh is currently seeking partners and funding to explore the feasibility of the following:

- Collaboration with the Product (RED) Initiative partners to design products to dress the red mannequins, to display them, and to launch a regional or global red mannequin HIV and AIDS awareness campaign with the support and facilitation of the World Bank's contacts
- Coordination with local designers in Bangladesh to design products using the red ribbon motif
- Coordination with various individuals and production clusters that designers work closely with to identify vocational training and employment opportunities for former IDUs and to start production clusters for people living with HIV to facilitate their economic independence
- Replication of the economic rehabilitation model through collaboration with various private sector partners to employ higher numbers of former IDUs and populations at high risk.

Nari Unnayan Shakti

Project title: Reduction of Stigma and Discrimination on HIV/AIDS through Media Sensitization and Reporting in Bangladesh

Implementing organization: Nari Unnayan Shakti (Women's Power for Development, or NUS)

Location: 64 districts, including trainings in Barisal, Dhaka, Chittagong, Khulna, and Sylhet

Background

Program goals: To increase in-depth knowledge and understanding of HIV and stigma and of discrimination among journalists and to enhance journalists' skills in articulating this information in newspaper articles

Target audiences: Journalists and general public (readers of newspapers)

Primary approaches: Training, media (newspapers)

Description of intervention: During the first four months of the project, NUS gained the necessary clearance from the government and adapted relevant training materials for the Bangladesh context. These materials consisted of modules on the epidemiology of HIV, understanding and challenging HIV stigma and discrimination, and nonstigmatizing language and messaging. NUS also reprinted two existing booklets on HIV available in Bengali for distribution to trainees. NUS then sent expression of interest letters regarding the project to all registered, high-circulation newspapers, or "dailies," that distribute 10,000 or more copies a day. Of newspapers contacted, 70 percent responded to the letter with interest. NUS followed up directly with editors to ensure that they sent properly trained, competent journalists to participate in the training and that they would provide space for publishing articles on HIV, AIDS, and stigma.

Beginning in November 2008, the project conducted six trainings of two days each throughout the country, covering all 64 districts. The trainings, which were targeted to local journalists from mainly rural areas, were participatory in nature and provided opportunity for interaction and discussion with persons living with HIV as well as time to draft articles and receive critical feedback from senior journalists and editors. Each training began with a two-hour inaugural session, to which key stakeholders—including senior government officials, the police superintendent, the president of the local press club, civil society representatives, the program manager of the National AIDS/Sexually Transmitted Disease Programme, the Joint Secretary of Health and Family Welfare, and the press—were invited. During this session, presentations were given on the HIV epidemic in Bangladesh and the challenges posed by stigma and discrimination.

Following the training, participants were asked to submit copies of articles they had written about HIV, AIDS, and stigma and discrimination as well as articles they had published. NUS followed up with journalists to encourage article submission and, as an incentive, offered certificates to those who submitted articles. These articles were entered into a competition. The top three stories were selected on the basis of article structure, factual content, and appropriate discussion of stigma in the context of HIV. Senior media representatives, including the head of a national television station and two editors of national newspapers, judged the competition. The winners were recognized in an awards ceremony on World AIDS Day at the culmination of the project.

Implementation, Results, and Challenges

Measurement strategy: Project monitoring

Results, key findings, and lessons: Overall, 288 journalists and other stakeholders participated in the inaugural sessions for the six trainings, and

137 local journalists were trained. By the end of the project period, 50 percent of local journalists trained had published articles in their local newspapers.

The participatory training sessions facilitated interaction between people living with HIV and journalists. Journalists overcame their own fears and misconceptions, and the trainings helped them understand the stigma and discrimination that people living with HIV face. Once their perceptions had shifted, the journalists were better equipped to address stigma and discrimination in their writing.

The trainings were also beneficial for the people living with HIV who participated and the networks of HIV-positive individuals they represented. The training provided an opportunity for the networks in three regions to link with journalists and local government officials, which may lead to more strategic engagement with local government and the media in the future.

The involvement of key stakeholders, such as national and local government officials, police officers, and members of civil society, from the onset of the project and in the inaugural events also contributed to the success of the project. Having clear support from senior-level government officials added credibility to the trainings, which helped draw journalists from high-circulation dailies to participate in the training and attracted more press coverage for the training events.

Challenges and unforeseen outcomes: Many of the articles written by trainees focused solely on HIV transmission and prevention and did not specifically address stigma and discrimination. Trainees also tended to focus on sexual transmission rather than other modes, such as needle sharing, that are common in Bangladesh.

Local journalists typically lack formal training and experience, which poses a challenge in developing trainings to strengthen their capacity. The lack of formal training and experience among the training participants was evident to the judges who selected the winning articles.

Additional Information

Program references, media coverage, and materials developed:

- Training curriculum
- Booklet on HIV and AIDS
- Stories about the project on 11 television stations after the initial inaugural workshop and in all high-circulation newspapers in Bangladesh

Contact information: Afroja Parvin, nusbdwomen@yahoo.com

Additional funding, replication, or scale-up opportunities or new partnerships resulting from the project: A stigma reduction network developed among journalists, with 130 members in six divisions of Bangladesh.

CHAPTER 14

India

Ashodaya Samithi

Project title: Addressing Stigma and Discrimination towards HIV+ Sex Workers and Sex Workers in General through Entrepreneurship

Implementing organization: Ashodaya Samithi

Location: Mysore

Background

Program goals: To (a) create a neutralizing environment and promote access to and use of health services by sex workers (including sex workers living with HIV) in public hospitals; (b) provide testimonies in social gatherings, media, and agencies to promote better understanding of HIV-positive life to garner greater support; (c) enhance the social position of sex workers (including sex workers living with HIV) through an economic enterprise that provides products for the mainstream; (d) educate the sex worker community on stigma and discrimination; and (e) document episodes of stigma and discrimination and measure decreases in stigma

Target audiences: Sex workers, government health professionals, police officers, and the general public

Primary approaches: Training, opening a business enterprise, advocacy, and support

Description of intervention: All activities were designed, planned, and implemented by sex workers, including sex workers living with HIV. The intervention had four components:

- Training sex workers in advocacy, with a focus on recognizing and addressing stigma and discrimination and on recognizing proper procedures and rights within the hospital. The project placed 20 trained sex workers (community guides) within eight health care facilities in Mysore to guide and support sex workers attending the facility and to sensitize health care workers.
- Training 15 sex workers living with HIV as social champions to provide testimonials of their personal experiences with learning their HIV status and living with HIV. Social champions took turns providing testimonials during workshops and meetings of various government and nongovernmental organizations, including outreach and advocacy with the local police force in Mysore.
- Forming and legally registering a support group by and for HIV-positive sex workers. The group originally met once a week but over time met just once a month. Following the support group meetings, participants were sensitized about stigma and discrimination through testimonials by senior sex worker community leaders, who shared their experiences with stigma. During these discussions, participants often shared their own experiences of stigma and discrimination. Where possible, community guides took actions to resolve these incidents.
- Opening a restaurant that employs sex workers to prepare and serve meals to the general public as an enterprise to generate income. The restaurant has expanded into catering various functions for local government authorities.

Implementation, Results, and Challenges

Measurement strategies: Process and monitoring data, including numbers trained, clients supported in health care settings, health care workers sensitized, number of cases of stigma and discrimination reported and resolved, and success of the restaurant in attracting customers

Results, key findings, and lessons: A key result was the successful positioning of volunteers in health care settings with total acceptance from health care providers as well as peripheral staff members. Sex workers found hospital staff members more sensitive and attentive to their needs when they were accompanied by the volunteers. Overall, 65 health personnel were sensitized. By the end of the project, 1,553 sex workers had accessed services in the government health care settings. Among these, 610 sex workers living with HIV were assisted for specific services such as registration for antiretroviral therapy (ART), CD4 count, x-rays, tuberculosis screening, and other blood tests.

To ensure the protection of the sex workers' rights, Ashodaya engaged with the police from the inception of the project. Recognizing that police officers are often transferred to other locations, Ashodaya conducted continuous advocacy, even becoming involved in cadet training. As a result, sex workers experienced reduced violence from the police during the project period. In addition, the police commissioner agreed to inaugurate the restaurant, representing a public statement of support for the sex worker community. This support led to more business for the restaurant in terms of dine-in customers and catering requests from government offices throughout Mysore and helped strengthen the sustainability of the restaurant and thus the care and support services provided to the community by Ashodaya. The restaurant typically serves more than 400 people a day, including government officials, students, and members of the general public. The social champions also engaged a number of additional stakeholders through 23 meetings and trainings conducted by Ashodaya for police personnel, conductors and drivers of Karnataka State Road Transport Corporation, and members of the Rotary Club.

Overall, 1,800 sex workers were sensitized about HIV stigma and discrimination. Project monitoring data showed that following the sensitization meetings, the number of incidents of discrimination reported by sex workers increased from 0 cases to 157. In 75 percent of these cases, a solution satisfactory to the aggrieved party was achieved. Narratives captured from sex worker community members suggested the increase in reporting occurred for two main reasons: (a) increased awareness of stigma and discrimination and (b) witnessing of the actions taken against the incidents. These two factors made the community more open to reporting incidents.

Challenges and unforeseen outcomes: This project has had several challenges and solutions. Every time a change occurs in police rank and file, Ashodaya meets with the new police officer to introduce the organization and to ask the officer to be a supportive partner of Ashodaya in preventing HIV transmission. Constant interaction with the community through awareness campaigns contributes to the visibility of sex workers (including sex workers with HIV) and the issues they face. A chef was hired to manage the restaurant, but the sex workers employed there are learning food preparation and restaurant management. Eventually sex workers will independently manage the entire operation of the restaurant from food preparation to staff and financial management.

Additional Information
Program references, media coverage, and materials developed:

- A short film, *Waves of Change*
- A photo book published to highlight HIV-positive living
- A report of Ashodaya's activities on CNNibn Web site: http://ibnlive .in.com/news/hotel-run-by-sex-workers-becomes-popular-in-mysore/83717-3-1.html
- Coverage about the restaurant on several news sites, summarized at http://www.indiaenews.com/pdf/164756.pdf

Contact information: Akram Pasha, ashodayasamithi@yahoo.co.in

Additional funding, replication, or scale-up opportunities or new partnerships resulting from the project: As a result of the project, Ashodaya has formed two new collaborations: one with an agency working with HIV-positive sex workers, Ashraya, and the other with the police to ensure protection of rights among sex workers. The government has recognized the value of the community guide volunteers in the health setting, and discussions are currently under way to sustain the participation of these volunteers. Several establishments have come forward to support Ashodaya's restaurant. For example, the Mysore City Corporation is working out details for catering services to its office, HSBC Bank has asked Ashodaya to cater food for all its office functions and meetings, a local college has hired Ashodaya to provide food to its students on special occasions, and the District Administration orders food from the restaurant on occasions such as World AIDS Day.

Development Initiative

Project title: Fighting Discrimination amongst the Population Suffering Most from the Prejudices Attached to HIV/AIDS

Implementing organizations: Development Initiative, Aident–Social Welfare Organisation, Our India

Location: Muzaffarpur railway station

Background

Program goals: To share knowledge about HIV, create empathy for people living with HIV, and raise awareness about the rights and services available to people living with HIV in the city of Muzaffarpur in Bihar, India

Target audience: General population (especially migrant laborers and railway station workers)

Primary approach: Outreach

Description of intervention: The Development Initiative implemented an awareness-raising project at the main railway station in Muzaffarpur and targeted railway station workers, including vendors, porters, rickshaw pullers, and police. Information gathered from initial interviews with railway staff members helped form an overall project strategy.

As part of the project, a television (TV) was installed in the railway station, and audiovisual material from the National AIDS Control Organisation (NACO) in India was shown on the TV. The audiovisual materials included testimonials of people living with HIV and information on HIV transmission. An audio program was also broadcast in the station using the TV speakers. People working in the station formed a street theater group and a folk ballad group. The project conducted six training sessions of two hours each to train people in street theater. The folk ballads and dramas took place on the platform and in three main trains (to Delhi, Kolkata, and Mumbai).

Implementation, Results, and Challenges

Measurement strategy: Qualitative data were collected through focus group discussions and key informant interviews. Initial key informant interviews were held with 100 vendors, porters, rickshaw pullers, and taxi drivers. A total of 20 focus group discussions with 10 to 12 people each were conducted at the project initiation and toward the end of the project. Overall, 70 railway staff members participated in focus group discussions. The project held four separate focus group discussions with the leaders of the porters and vendors, lower-level railway workers, senior functionaries of the railway station, and rickshaw pullers and auto drivers.

Results, key findings, and lessons: Ultimately, 25 people working around the railway station were trained in street theater, and they put on 140 street theater performances with themes revolving around stigma and discrimination associated with HIV. The folk ballad group put on 50 folk dance performances with interwoven traditional stories.

A major success of the project was the sensitization of the railway station workers. The project helped raise awareness among them about different aspects of HIV and associated stigma and discrimination. Previously, even to mention the word *condom* in a place like the Muzaffarpur station was taboo, but now porters and hawkers are distributing condoms to people coming through the station and talking to the public about HIV. As a result of the project, a solid peer group of 125 railway station workers exists that will be the backbone of all the future programs. In terms of the broader reach of project activities among the general public, the project estimates that approximately 4,000 people move through the railway station every day with the potential opportunity to engage in program activities.

The focus group discussions conducted at the project's inception revealed people's great reluctance to talk about HIV and AIDS. Focus group participants seemed to think that people living with HIV "got what they deserved." The focus group discussions conducted toward the end of the project revealed a positive shift in people's perceptions about HIV and AIDS and related stigma and discrimination.

Challenges and unforeseen outcomes: A major challenge was initially connecting with railway staff members and generating interest among them to participate in the project. Because the station serves hundreds of trains and thousands of commuters every day, drawing the attention and the time of the workers was difficult. This challenge was addressed by approaching the leaders of the railway staff, conducting an initial meeting with them, and then expanding the meetings to the entire railway staff. The meetings were held at a time of day when more staff members were likely to be available.

Additional Information
Program references, media coverage, and materials developed: The project used existing information, education, and communication (IEC) and training materials for project activities.

Contact information: Sanjay Kumar, sanjay@developmentinitiative.org; kjsanjay@gmail.com

Additional funding, replication, or scale-up opportunities or new partnerships resulting from the project: NACO has agreed to continue to fund the program at Muzaffarpur station. Also, partly because it is a South Asia Region Development Marketplace (SARDM) recipient, the Development Initiative is currently partnering with NACO to produce radio programs for All India Radio. The content of the radio programs largely focuses on awareness about HIV and AIDS and discrimination in community settings, the workplace, health care settings, and schools.

ISTV Network

Project title: Fighting Discrimination through Awareness: Game Show

Implementing organizations: ISTV Network, Institute of Social Work and Research

Location: ISTV Network, Gambhir Singh Shopping Arcade, Bir Tikendrajit Road, Imphal, Manipur

Background

Program goals: To create general awareness of HIV and AIDS, help decrease stigma and discrimination associated with HIV and AIDS, and bring about attitude change toward people living with HIV through the game show *Get the Facts, Make a Difference by Reducing Stigma*

Target audience: General population

Primary approach: Game show

Description of intervention: The project produced and aired a game show in Manipur, India, featuring information and awareness-raising on HIV and AIDS–related stigma and discrimination. Shows were aired four times a week. The show had a host, two contestants, and 25 guests in the audience during each show. Episodes were recorded ahead of time rather than aired live. Contestants sat in the "hot seat" and responded to questions posed by the host. The contestant who pressed the buzzer first answered the question. Correct answers received Rs 300, and incorrect answers led to the loss of Rs 100. The grand prize at the end of the year was a new car.

Initially, the project selected contestants from among the studio audience through an audience questionnaire. The two top scorers were selected as contestants for that episode. After 13 episodes, selection switched to a written competition (500 people responded) to select the 38 contestants for the remaining 16 episodes.

Questions for each episode were developed with support from the World Bank and local experts in HIV and AIDS such as staff from the Manipur State AIDS Control Society and local nongovernmental organizations (NGOs).

Experts were present during the show to provide more expansive information and clarification on the questions being asked, and they were available after the show to interact with the audience, answering more questions. These experts included the former director of the Manipur AIDS Control Society. People living with HIV or others who have faced stigma or discrimination answered questions related to stigma and discrimination.

Five special episodes involving only individuals living with HIV were recorded and aired. The Manipur Network of People living with HIV assisted in developing special questions for these episodes, and NGO representatives and other stakeholders served as experts. The host hugged and shook hands with contestants in an effort to reinforce the message that HIV is not transmitted through casual contact and reduce stigma and discrimination against people living with HIV. A special episode for media personnel and one for Manipur-based employees of Aircel, a mobile phone company, were also produced. One episode featured famous film stars as contestants in the hot seat.

Implementation, Results, and Challenges

Measurement strategies: An end-line survey was conducted among 3,000 ISTV viewers across the four districts covered by the ISTV network. The project selected viewers by identifying houses with an ISTV cable network connection. The survey questionnaire was administered by trained field investigators and sampled specific target groups: 1,000 housewives, 1,500 students, 200 employees, 200 people living with HIV, 200 doctors and nurses working in the field of HIV, and 50 lawyers.

Structured one-on-one interviews with a set of determined questions were conducted with 30 game show participants (five participants were chosen from each of the first six episodes) to assess their perception of the show and whether they thought they gained knowledge of HIV. Individual interviews were also done with viewers, including HIV experts, service providers, students, and housewives.

The Institute of Social Work and Research conducted participant evaluations with 30 participants who had been selected for the hot seat and with 30 invited audience members.

Focus groups were conducted with 11 groups of NGO representatives working in the field of HIV and AIDS, with a group of people living with HIV, and with a group of graduate-level students.

Results, key findings, and lessons: A total of 68 episodes were aired across four districts to an estimated half million viewers.

Of end-line survey respondents, 67 percent said they would be willing to participate in the game show, and more than half of viewers surveyed (53 percent) reported watching the show regularly. Most viewers discussed the game show with friends (69 percent) and family members (72 percent). Nearly all viewers (90 percent) felt the game show was useful in educating viewers on HIV and AIDS, and 94 percent felt the game show would help reduce stigma and discrimination.

Of structured interview respondents, 96 percent said they gained new knowledge as a result of their participation. More than half (64 percent) were satisfied with the questions asked of the contestants and felt the questions allowed viewers to easily learn new information that will lead to reductions in stigma and discrimination. Almost all hot seat participants (95 percent of 120) reported studying and seeking information about HIV and AIDS from relevant books, visits to NGOs, doctors, and discussions with family and friends in preparation for being on the show.

The NGO representatives who participated in the focus groups received phone calls and personal visits from likely student participants, as well as their parents, seeking information on HIV and AIDS. NGOs with telephone counseling centers reported an increase in calls, and when the callers were asked the reason, the game show was given. The NGO focus group participants indicated the game show was an entertaining and informative way of engaging housewives who have limited access to other external educational materials. The NGO focus group participants also found the game show questions informative because they contained knowledge, showed a positive attitude, and provided details on services and the treatment process.

One filmmaker, inspired by the game show, shot an episode with Manipur's favorite actors, Sadananda and Raju, in the hot seat. In the storyline, Sadananda marries an HIV-positive woman because of the knowledge he gained in participating in the *Get the Facts, Make a Difference by Reducing Stigma* game show.

Challenges and unforeseen outcomes: The initial contestant selection process proved time consuming, and getting 25 audience members at each show was a challenge. After 13 episodes, the selection process was changed to a written competition, which allowed a larger and more diverse group an opportunity to be on the show. Specific invitations were extended to special groups to be in the audience, including students and nurse trainees, to bring in more stakeholders and to confirm a full audience for each episode.

The law and order situation in Imphal (curfews, for example) and an erratic power supply also created a challenge. ISTV responded by having the print media print the questions following the telecasts so that people who missed the telecast would still know what questions were asked.

Additional Information

Program references, media coverage, and materials developed:

- Questionnaires for show
- Promos
- DVD recordings of all episodes

Contact information: Yumnam Rupachandra Singh, Project Manager, yumnamrupa@gmail.com

Lotus Integrated AIDS Awareness Sangam

Project title: Advocacy by Cultural Teams (ACT)

Implementing organization: Lotus Integrated AIDS Awareness Sangam

Location: Thanjavur, Nagapattinam, and Thiruvarur districts of Tamil Nadu

Background

Program goals: To use theater to change harmful attitudes and practices blocking the access of men who have sex with men (MSM) and transgender populations to entitlements and legal redress through their municipal governments, or panchayats

Target audiences: Village panchayats and community members

Primary approach: Theater

Description of intervention: Lotus undertook a careful process to develop and implement its theater intervention. It conducted focus group interviews with MSM and panchayat leaders to inform script development. A member of Lotus wrote the script. The implementation process also involved hiring a staff, securing and setting up office and performance practice space, contracting professional theater trainers, and holding auditions for the cultural team.

Lotus mobilized additional support from the Indian Network for People Living with HIV/AIDS (INP+) to intensify its work with panchayat leaders in performance villages. This effort entailed organizing two one-day trainings on HIV and AIDS, MSM, and transgender populations for panchayat leaders.

Lotus selected villages for the performances on the basis of its knowledge of where MSM resided and the willingness of the local panchayat leaders to have a performance in their community. Because Lotus had a letter of support from the Tamil Nadu State AIDS Control Society, its entry into villages was relatively smooth.

Implementation, Results, and Challenges

Measurement strategy: Focus group discussions were conducted at baseline and end line with MSM and with panchayat leaders.

Results, key findings, and lessons: Seventy-five performances were given in three districts. Each performance drew a crowd of approximately 150, with total audience members reaching an estimated 11,250.

The project achieved success in opening up a justice channel through panchayat leaders as well as in an array of unanticipated areas. Panchayat leaders reported changes in their attitudes and behaviors. The consensus among those interviewed was that although they thought 100 percent of panchayat leaders had understood the issues presented in the play, about 50 percent of leaders had an exceptionally strong positive reaction, actively demonstrating changes in behavior. Some panchayat leaders are actively seeking out MSM under their jurisdiction to talk with them, tell them about the play, and encourage them to visit Lotus offices.

Men who have sex with men confirmed positive changes in their lives, discussing how important the play was for them in recognizing that they were not alone, that there were others like them, and that there was a support group they could join. As of mid-December 2009, 147 "hidden" village MSM had approached the actors after a performance, and of these, 47 had visited the Lotus office, often at some distance from their villages, to seek support. Of these 47, 42 have accessed counseling services at Lotus, 19 were referred to a government hospital to be tested for HIV and sexually transmitted infections (STIs) and to receive treatment as required. Two MSM told Lotus that they were experiencing stigma and discrimination from local men (being forced to have sex and being threatened for money as well as teased in public) and asked for support to resolve these issues. These problems were successfully addressed by Lotus leaders, in one case with the help of a panchayat leader.

In addition, interview respondents reported seeing a drop in the harassment they face in public spaces, such as the market or taxi stands, as well as a new willingness by villagers to engage in normal, daily social interactions with them. Some had even received apologies from villagers for past behavior. Others reported how some villagers have stepped in to challenge teasing and harassment of MSM and transgender persons, something that never occurred before the play.

The intervention strengthened Lotus's capacity in project management, as well as its ability to use theater, improve the health and well-being of its clients, and secure additional funds.

Challenges and unforeseen outcomes: At two performances, some audience members arrived intoxicated and disrupted the performance. In response, future performances were scheduled in venues away from wine shops.

During election season, panchayat leaders sometimes used the events to further their own political agendas. To counter personal political agendas, performances were scheduled well in advance of elections.

The implementing organization had to work around monsoon season to complete performances on schedule.

Additional Information
Program references, media coverage, and materials developed:

- Script of play
- Four evaluation reports on baseline and end-line data
- Calendar developed for stakeholders
- Film titled *Justice of the Mute*, which documents a performance with audience reaction
- Feature article highlighting the play by *Nakeeran*, a Tamilian biweekly journal with a wide readership (September 2009)
- Coverage of Lotus and the play in the local Kumbakonam press three times (May, June, and November 2009)
- Documentation of the play by an independent international photojournalist

Contact information: N. Muthukumar, lotus_sangam@yahoo.co.in

Additional funding, replication, or scale-up opportunities or new partnerships resulting from the project: As a result of the project, Lotus Sangam has achieved growing recognition at the local, district, and state levels in India, as well as internationally. Lotus is now a member of a national transgender convening committee supported by the United Nations Development Programme and has also received support from INP+ to conduct trainings and participate in local and state-level events. Lotus now participates in important meetings and events in Tamil Nadu dealing with issues of concern to MSM and transgender persons.

Lotus is also a founding organization, along with three other community organizations in Tamil Nadu, for a state-level forum, the United Network of MSM Advocacy and AIDS Initiatives (UNMAAI—in Tamil, this means truth or fact). At the local level, panchayats have invited Lotus representatives to attend village events. Lotus has also received several international visitors seeking information on the project and was hired by an international researcher to conduct field interviews, which took place in January 2010.

Nalandaway Foundation

Project title: Nalandaway Children Media Project

Implementing organization: Nalandaway Foundation

Location: Tamil Nadu

Background
Program goals: To provide a platform for adults to learn the difficulties that HIV-positive children undergo by helping HIV-infected and affected children and youth share through film the incidents of discrimination, fear, and stigma that they have experienced

Target audience: General population

Primary approaches: Training, film

Description of intervention: This project is informing a documentary to showcase the stigma and discrimination faced by children living with and affected by HIV. The forthcoming film is intended to increase knowledge and shift attitudes among the public through public screenings in cinemas and on TV.

This intervention involved a participatory training workshop for children to develop a script on stigma reduction, followed by further script development by professional scriptwriters. The project used a talent search to identify children seven to 17 years of age to participate in the workshop. The children, some of whom were HIV-positive or affected by HIV, were selected from secondary schools, care homes, and orphanages and through World Vision programs.

Implementation, Results, and Challenges
Measurement strategies: The project used qualitative baseline research to investigate stigma and discrimination in various communities in Tamil Nadu. Key informant interviews were conducted with people in

school management, teachers, children (both in and out of school), hospital staff members (medical and nonmedical), and landlords. The interviews attempted to assess knowledge levels of modes of HIV transmission and attitudes toward HIV-infected children. In all, the project interviewed 175 people and collected 19 case studies from networks of people living with HIV around Tamil Nadu that support children who are living with or affected by HIV. The networks include the Shelter Foundation.

In addition to the key informant interviews, the project team conducted a baseline survey with teachers, school managers, parent-teacher association presidents, school staff members, schoolchildren, and medical and nonmedical hospital staff.

The film release will be followed by an impact assessment involving group discussions and in-depth interviews with those who have seen the film.

Results, key findings, and lessons: Findings from the baseline survey revealed the following:

- More than 50 percent of school management personnel were not familiar with the modes of HIV transmission.
- Almost 80 percent of respondents did not know the difference between HIV and AIDS.
- Less than 20 percent of hospital staff members were willing to treat an HIV-positive patient.
- Of headmasters, 60 percent were hesitant to admit an HIV-positive child to their school.
- Of the children interviewed, 30 percent were scared to play with an HIV-positive child.

The project trained 30 children in a 10-day participatory workshop in creative thinking, drama, photography, music, storytelling, and filmmaking. The children were asked to create a script on stigma reduction, and professional scriptwriters further developed the script.

This project informed the film, which is under way. The project team anticipates the film will be an initial catalyst sparking further discussion and action in the community.

Challenges and unforeseen outcomes: During the talent search, rejecting children from further participation was challenging. To ease disappointment, these children were given an opportunity to participate in other art projects.

Additional Information

Program references, media coverage, and materials developed:

- Scripts and stories written by the children participating in the project
- Storyboard developed by children and professionals for the feature film
- Workshop report
- Model film written and directed by children
- Test shoot of the feature film

Contact information: Sriram Ayer, sriram@nalandaway.org

Additional funding, replication, or scale-up opportunities or new partnerships resulting from the project: Nalandaway has secured the partnership of two large production houses: Real Image Media Technologies (http://www.realimage.com/) and Sathyam Cinemas (http://www.sathyamcinemas.com/). These production houses have agreed to provide funding to make the film, providing state-of-the-art technology and production values, and distribute it to more than 250 screens across the state of Tamil Nadu for at least 50 days. This distribution should reach a large general public, including opinion leaders. Premium channel Star Vijay TV will also screen the film, thereby reaching audiences who missed it in theaters.

Sai Paranjpye Films

Project title: Qisse (Episodes)

Implementing organization: Sai Paranjpye Films

Location: Sanjay Gandhi Transport Nagar (New Delhi) and Nigdi (Pune, Maharashtra)

Background

Program goals: To develop short films to reduce HIV and AIDS–related stigma and discrimination in an innovative way

Target audiences: Marginalized groups including sex workers and their clients (truckers), injecting drug users, organizations working with these groups, and the general public

Primary approach: Filmmaking

Description of intervention: Sai Paranjpye Films researched and produced two films for its project titled *Qisse* (episodes in English). *Suee* (*The Needle*) is a 29-minute film featuring a series of personal narratives of the lives and experiences of drug users in Mumbai. The script for *Suee* was developed in collaboration with two prominent NGOs, Sharan in New Delhi and Sankalp in Mumbai. Both NGOs provide services in drug rehabilitation, HIV risk awareness and prevention, and hepatitis C prevention and treatment. The project also consulted former drug users turned activists. The team developed scripts in November and December 2008. The scripts featured a dramatic storyline that drew on the lives of actual drug users, making this film a unique blend of fiction and reality. Social workers, doctors and medical workers, outreach workers, and drug users from Sankalp appear in the film. The film was shot entirely in Mumbai with the cooperation and encouragement of the commissioner of police and the inspector general of prisons. Several scenes in the film were shot in a police cell and in a prison.

The second film, *Horrn Pukare* (*Call of the Horn*), is a 24-minute film shot in several locations, including highways; the Sanjay Gandhi Transport Nagar company; and the transport town of Nigdi, Maharashtra. The film illustrates the risks faced by truck drivers in the context of HIV and AIDS. The process of developing *Horrn Pukare* entailed consultation and discussion starting in July 2008 with the Transport Corporation of India and among truckers and workers at the Sanjay Gandhi Transport Nagar and in the transport town of Nigdi in Maharashtra.

The team gathered a great deal of information in preparing the film; the original 6-minute short film planned turned into a 24-minute film. The filmmaker, Sai Paranjpye, consulted with the AIDS Prevention and Control Project of Tamil Nadu, the National AIDS Control Programme, and the AIDS Research Control Centre for information, input, and advice. The completed script was reviewed and discussed with truck drivers in numerous meetings and group sessions to ensure that it reflected the lifestyles, problems, and experiences of trucker drivers in the context of HIV and AIDS.

Implementation, Results, and Challenges
Measurement strategy: Track demand for the films postproduction

Results, key findings, and lessons: The response to both films has been great. The launch was attended by many well-known government officials as well as international and social service groups. Both films received excellent press reviews.

Suee debuted in India in Mumbai on July 2, 2009, and was hosted by the Narcotics Control Bureau at the American Center. The film was also shown at the International Conference on AIDS in Asia and the Pacific in Bali, Indonesia, on July 8, 2009, and at the International Harm Reduction Association's 21st International Conference in Liverpool, United Kingdom, in April 2010. The film has been acquired by several NGOs and other organizations for screening among their members, including Air Headquarters, Anand Foundation, Johnson & Johnson, Muktangan, Narcotics Control Bureau, Sangram Sangli, Sankalp Drug Rehabilitation Foundation, Sharan and Humana People to People Foundation, and Tata Motors.

The film *Horrn Pukare* is being shown throughout the truck drivers' networks through the Transport Corporation of India, and screenings are followed by workshops and interactive sessions with facilitators. A local organization in Nigdi shows the film regularly as part of its HIV and AIDS awareness drives. ICICI Bank and the Mehandale Transport Group of Pune also show the film during workshops. An English subtitled version appears on the World Bank Web site, and DVDs of the film have been sent to the AIDS Prevention and Control project in Tamil Nadu, the Mumbai Districts AIDS Control Society, and the National AIDS Control Programme.

Challenges and unforeseen outcomes: A controversial scene in the film *Suee*, where two inmates discuss condom use, had to be adapted by the filmmaker because of sensitivities to the existence of men having sex with men in prisons. In collaboration with prison authorities, the script sequence was changed to inmates being trained for "after-release eventualities."

Additional Information
Program references, media coverage, and materials developed: Two films, *Suee* and *Horrn Pukare*

Contact information: Sai Paranjpye, saiparanjpye@gmail.com

Additional funding, replication, or scale-up opportunities or new partnerships resulting from the project: The Transport Corporation of India helped to make *Horrn Pukare* a credible exercise through research, access, script development, and evaluation. *Suee* was similarly supported by the Sankalp Drug Rehabilitation Trust.

Saral

Project title: Food and Catering Services for PLHA

Implementing organizations: Saral in collaboration with Aadhar

Location: Ahmedabad, Gujarat

Background

Program goals: Saral, in partnership with Aadhar (a network of people living with HIV in Ahmedabad, Gujarat, India), initiated a project to provide people living with HIV opportunities to work in food production and distribution, thus reducing stigma and discrimination.

Target audiences: General population and people living with HIV and AIDS

Primary approach: Employment

Description of intervention: The food program focused on involving people living with HIV from Aadhar in catering services as well as distribution of dry snacks. The Aadhar Mahila Trust (AMT) was formed to manage the SARDM grant and to enable Aadhar to get involved with commercial activities. AMT's mission included creating income-generating activities, providing a platform for women living with HIV, and giving legal guidance.

On the basis of a needs assessment, the project team developed trainings for the trustees and board members of AMT, the Saral team, the food production team, and the outreach team. The topics covered in the trainings included marketing techniques, team building and leadership, food production and hospitality management, business development and entrepreneurship, community-based organization management, nutritious cooking, and ways to establish links with Aadhar's existing drop-in centers.

AMT provided packed snacks at the civil hospital canteen, the Apna Bazar, and the State Bank of India canteen. AMT initially faced challenges finding volunteers, developing local leadership, and working with different NGOs. AMT decided to provide food for work at the drop-in center, where eight to 10 people eat on a daily basis, as an incentive for volunteers involved in the distribution of snack packets and catering events. The location was next to the district civil hospital, so people coming for ART could stop in for food.

Implementation, Results, and Challenges
Measurement strategy:

- Project monitoring was done through process indicators, including terms of reference and system development for the Governance and Management Committee; meetings of the Governance and Management Committee; terms of reference and systems establishment for the food production facilities; procurement of space for food production; identification of team for catering services, training, and capacity development of team; and establishment of a supportive supervision structure.
- Interviews with project participants were conducted at the end of the project.

Results, key findings, and lessons: One significant achievement was the opportunity to create an identity for AMT and for HIV-positive women involved in social-profit activities. Additional outcomes included the provision of dignified options for people living with HIV who needed to make a sustainable living and the development of a strong relationship with the Ahmedabad Municipal Corporation for establishing distribution channels and legal processes related to food production and services. The project established a full-fledged food production center. In addition, the project trained a team of 12 members identified for the food production center in Aadhar and arranged for a mobile food van (donated by the State Bank of India) to provide food services to the entire city. A key outcome was that the confidence and enthusiasm of the members involved in the project from Aadhar have gradually increased, as is apparent in their food marketing efforts and their adoption of these activities as sustainable livelihood options.

Project participants reported changes in their lives, such as more optimistic mind-sets, increased respect from spouses and family members, reduction of stigma and discrimination, higher self-esteem, and increased capacities for sustainable livelihood (four HIV-positive people have started their own businesses with seed capital funding from Aadhar and Saral). All involved now want to continue work in the project on a full-time basis.

Challenges and unforeseen outcomes: The food supply activities—supplying catering for events and selling dry packed food through street stands or booths and door-to-door sales—turned out to be a slow-growing business. About 50 people living with HIV worked in snack distribution (sales stands and door-to-door sales). The people engaged in selling the food packets were unable to work full time and were worried about exposing their status. Having enough personnel available for cooking and producing the dry snacks was a challenge. As a result, a subcontractor was hired to produce the dry snacks, which were in turn packed by people living with HIV and sold door to door by another group of volunteers. Toward the end of the project, the team had addressed the personnel challenges. Ten full-time, fully trained HIV-positive women will attend the central kitchen. Auto drivers and mobile sellers have been appointed.

Additional Information
Program references, media coverage, and materials developed: The project received significant media attention and interest. TV, radio, and print media all covered various project activities. Media covering project activities included Dur Darshan, All India Radio, Radio 91.1 FM, Radio Mirchi, *Times of India, Ahmedabad Mirror, Gujarat Samachar, Divya Bhaskar, Sandesh,* and *Rajasthan Patrika.* The project carried out about eight folk media performances based on a script developed on stigma and discrimination, and 2,000 people attended the performances. At least 40 media people are now familiar with AMT and its activities and the Food for Work project.

Contact information: Hemalee Leuva, hemalee@ramanagroup.org

Additional funding, replication, or scale-up opportunities or new partnerships resulting from the project: The State Bank of India donated a mobile van for food. The Adani Foundation contributed to remodeling and equipping the van. The Employees' State Insurance Corporation provided subsidized space for a central kitchen in the heart of Ahmedabad. The wholesale grain merchants association contributed 100 kilograms of wheat and 50 kilograms of rice. The Entrepreneurship Development Institute, Ahmedabad Management Association, International Center for Entrepreneurship and Career Development, Home Science Department of B.D. Arts College, Akshay Patra Foundation, and ATI School of Leadership Development contributed through high (up to 50 percent) subsidization of training and capacity-building costs. Ten postgraduate students of social welfare contributed by helping with project activities as needed. Opinion leaders such as Mallika Sarabhai expressed their support by appearing on AMT's promotional brochures free of cost. Raman Development Consultants announced a donation for taking the project ahead and buying equipment for preparing hot and fresh snacks. Several agencies have come forward to offer outlets. The Ahmedabad Municipal Corporation has committed to provide an outlet at Kankaria Lake. Adani Foundation and Digvijay Lions Foundation supported school fees, uniforms, textbooks, notebooks, and schoolbags for 300 children affected by or living with HIV. Nagraj Gruh Udhyog, Sadvichar Parivar, Smart Namkin, and Vishal Chavana all contributed by subsidizing their prices of dry snacks for AMT up to 25 percent of their prevailing rates.

AMT envisions continuing the project, building on the foundation established. A new menu has been designed on the basis of advisory inputs of the Home Science Department, B.D. Arts College. Advocacy with Ahmedabad Municipal Corporation has provided hawkers with licenses for promising junctions. The Employees' State Insurance Corporation has asked AMT to consider managing its staff canteen.

Society for Positive Atmosphere and Related Support to HIV/AIDS

Project title: Art and Testimonial: A Unique Community-Based Approach to Reduce HIV/AIDS Stigma in Villages of West Bengal

Implementing organizations: Society for Positive Atmosphere and Related Support to HIV/AIDS (SPARSHA), in partnership with MAKE ART/STOP AIDS and National Institute of Cholera and Enteric Diseases (Indian Council of Medical Research)

Location: Paschim Medinipur and Howrah districts, in the state of West Bengal in eastern India

Background

Program goals: To change negative attitudes of communities toward people living with HIV, to reduce the impact of stigma and discrimination toward adults living with HIV, to ensure sustainability of intervention efforts, and to create a supportive environment in schools where HIV-affected children study

Target audiences: General population and people living with HIV

Primary approaches: Community engagement, solidarity between people living with HIV and those not infected with HIV, traditional music and dance, and outreach

Description of intervention: The project was implemented in two distinct phases. The first half of the 18-month period entailed active involvement of project staff members in planning and executing the intervention in consultation with community members. The latter half was characterized by gradual takeover of activities by community members. The six elements of this intervention were (a) community engagement, (b) formation of a stigma reduction committee, (c) creation of a team of community health workers (CHWs) comprising people living with HIV and those not infected with HIV who worked together and thus created a role model, (d) music and dance performance by the local artists paired with discussion about HIV steered by CHWs in communities and schools, (e) assistance to school authorities and teachers in drafting a declaration on nondiscriminatory practice protecting the rights of children, and (f) outreach to families with someone living with HIV to address various unmet needs.

The project randomly selected four control and four intervention villages. At the start of the project, a baseline assessment was conducted in all eight villages. The intervention used a traditional form of music and dance (Baul and Tarja) to engage community members in discussions of HIV prevention, care and treatment, and stigma and discrimination. In addition to these activities, the intervention consisted of three consecutive performances by Baul singers, held once a week over a three-week period during the first nine months of the project. Each performance was dedicated to a specific topic. The first performance focused on how HIV is transmitted, the second focused on personal experiences of people living with HIV in the community and HIV prevention methods, and the third focused on care and support for people living with HIV. Before and after each performance, the HIV-positive CHW and HIV-negative district team leader led a group discussion with community members who gathered for the performance. This forum allowed community members to ask questions and also provided a chance for them to interact with a person living openly with HIV. The Baul singers, who were mostly farmers, performed in a group wearing traditional saffron-colored cloaks and played different musical instruments, sang, and danced. They worked with the project staff, including people living with HIV, to develop the song lyrics they performed. The performances were repeated once in the second phase of the project.

Implementation, Results, and Challenges

Measurement strategies: The project followed an experimental design (using indicators from the International Center for Research on Women's work in Tanzania and from the Joint United Nations Programme on HIV/AIDS). A baseline assessment was conducted that included one-on-one interviews, focus group discussions, in-depth interviews, and key informant interviews.

Additional funding was secured to organize sessions to provide input for the local performing artists (Baul and Tarja singers) and to assist in assessing the effectiveness of the intervention. An assessment is currently under way that uses both qualitative and quantitative data analysis techniques.

Results, key findings, and lessons: Overall, the project had a number of positive outcomes. For example, stigma reduction committees, which are joint initiatives of people living with HIV and community members, were formed and are encouraging nondiscriminatory practices at the community level. One of the committees decided to address issues of stigma when an incident of discrimination occurring in a neighboring village came to its attention. Another important outcome was that the project linked people living with HIV in the intervention areas to opportunities and services they could access, including generating income, receiving various treatment services, and at times even ensuring vaccination or education support for their children through outreach and advocacy with appropriate health and school authorities.

Using traditional music and dance as the mode of message delivery seemed to affect community members powerfully and was well received by the members living with HIV and their families. Positive changes in attitudes among community members in the villages of the intervention arm were clearly articulated by people living with HIV interviewed after the intervention. Neighbors who closely witnessed the interaction of the project staff members and artists with people living with HIV and their families have proactively started mixing socially again with those families. In addition, school authorities in the intervention arm drafted a declaration on nondiscriminatory practices with regard to education and psychosocial development of children. The Baul singers mentioned that following the intervention, communities requested the troupe to sing the HIV- and stigma-related songs during their performances at community events unrelated to the project. This phenomenon indicates the popularity of the songs developed and suggests longer-lasting exposure to the HIV songs and messages after the intervention.

The results of the analysis thus far suggest that implementing a stigma reduction program on the basis of the six-element intervention package described previously is effective and therefore worth the resources. If well planned and executed, programs do not take a prohibitively long time to produce results. However, different sources of stigma in the community do not change equally to exposure of intervention, and this issue requires further research.

Challenges and unforeseen outcomes: One of the village sites initially objected to parts of the performance focusing on HIV. After discussions with religious and political leaders, the performance was allowed at a site in one of the intervention villages.

Additional Information

Program references, media coverage, and materials developed: Materials developed include the following:

- A print publication, *Art and Public Health: Report on Development of a Unique Community-Based Approach to Reduce HIV/AIDS Stigma in Villages of West Bengal*
- A documentary DVD with two short films (one of three minutes and another of eight minutes).

These items may be used for advocacy aiming to translate research findings into action. Articles to be published on the project findings will add to this effort.

Contact information: Samiran Panda, dr.samiran_panda@rediffmail.com

Additional funding, replication, or scale-up opportunities or new partnerships resulting from the project: Additional funding from Princess Diana Foundation and Ford Foundation helped in organizing sessions to provide input for local artists (Baul and Tarja singers) and to fine-tune the artistic components of the intervention.

Institutional support from the National Institute of Cholera and Enteric Diseases, a permanent institute of the Indian Council of Medical Research located in Kolkata, West Bengal, played a key role in assessing the effect of the project.

Random allocation of clusters by drawing lots in the intervention and control arms was carried out through the active participation of community opinion leaders and officials from the West Bengal State AIDS Prevention and Control Society. Future advocacy for a scaled-up response and an assessment of the effectiveness of the scaled intervention would require additional funding.

Swathi Mahila Sangha

Project title: Spoorthi: Community Action against Stigma and Discrimination: Project Baduku

Implementing organizations: Swathi Mahila Sangha, Vijaya Mahila Sangha, Jyothi Mahila Sangha, Swasti Health Resource Center, Bhoruka Charitable Trust

Location: All seven zones of Bangalore, Karnataka

Background

Program goals: To empower and build the capacity of women in sex work to challenge stigma and discrimination by leading advocacy efforts directed at the general public and key secondary stakeholders, such as police and health care workers, as well as the partners, family members, and neighbors of women in sex work. The campaigns sought to sensitize these populations about the issues faced by women in sex work and people living with HIV and to seek support to help change the attitudes and biases in society.

Target audiences: Female sex workers (including those living with HIV), the general public, key secondary stakeholders

Primary approaches: Leadership and stigma reduction training, advocacy campaigns and targeted advocacy

Description of intervention: The project began with formative research to inform the content of advocacy messages and to determine the target populations. The next step was to recruit and train the project staff, including 15 community mobilizers and a project coordinator. All staff members were women in sex work and most were HIV positive. The project provided women with leadership training and training on stigma and discrimination. Project staff members then went on to lead advocacy events, directly engaging secondary stakeholders and working with the families and neighbors of women in sex work to address reported cases of stigma and discrimination. In addition, the project team was actively engaged in capacity building and support efforts among women in sex work living with HIV.

The advocacy campaigns were designed to highlight the positive role that public and secondary stakeholders can play in improving the lives of women in sex work, rather than blaming them for the stigma and discrimination they experience as sex workers. The project used numerous strategies for engaging the public, such as the Signature campaign, the Human Chain campaign, and the Handshake campaign. Other campaigns were targeted specifically toward secondary stakeholders. In the Bike campaign, hundreds of women in sex work and supporters of the stigma reduction efforts rode to hospitals around the city to engage medical professionals in a discussion about the issues facing women in sex work living with HIV. The Rose campaign went a step further to recognize doctors and police officers who had been particularly supportive and sensitive to the sex worker community and to request their help in convincing their colleagues to do the same. Project staff members also presented roses to people who had been particularly stigmatizing and abusive in the past, to spur change head-on.

In addition to these advocacy campaigns, project staff members engaged in targeted advocacy as needed. For example, community mobilizers responded to specific cases of discrimination reported by female sex workers, including isolation by family members and avoidance by neighbors. The crisis response teams of the three support organizations were also trained to identify and respond to cases of discrimination. Last, the media were engaged strategically throughout the project to expand the reach of advocacy messages. The media were informed about the location and times of all public advocacy events to enhance press coverage.

Implementation, Results, and Challenges

Measurement strategy: Project monitoring and formative research were used to assess the level and main sources of stigma and discrimination among women in sex work.

The project staff developed an innovative pictorial questionnaire that could be implemented by female sex workers with minimal literacy skills. Data were collected from 166 women in sex work who were accessed at drop-in centers and in the field. The findings highlighted the need to address internalized stigma among women in sex work and sex workers living with HIV. In addition, the data identified key secondary stakeholders to target for advocacy.

Results, key findings, and lessons: More than 400 existing staff members from the three support organizations were trained on stigma and discrimination so they could participate in the various advocacy events held around the city.

In the health care setting, increases in the percentage of HIV-positive female sex workers regularly seeking care and treatment services at ART centers in Bangalore increased from 30 to 60 percent following the project. Women appeared to be more comfortable sharing their HIV status with their families and project staff members. Overall, health care workers perceived the campaign positively.

More than 221 campaigns were conducted throughout Bangalore, reaching over 2,150 secondary stakeholders. During the Signature campaign and other campaigns, 132,000 individuals signed and pledged not to stigmatize or discriminate against women in sex work. More than 225,000 were reached in the other campaigns.

The Rose campaign was particularly effective at reaching secondary stakeholders. Following the campaign, the number of cases of stigma and discrimination reported by female sex workers to the police grew from 0 to 11, all of which the police actively responded to and resolved. In addition, sex workers anecdotally reported less harassment and violence from police officers following the intervention in a jurisdiction where violence had previously been quite high.

The commitment of the HIV-positive women leading the project to proactively engage with stakeholders and try to improve their environment motivated many stakeholders to join with the women in support of their stigma reduction efforts. Strengthening the capacity of women in sex work living with HIV to lead stigma reduction efforts provided both motivation and inspiration. Many of the women reported new confidence and courage, which enabled them to confront stigma and discrimination in their own lives and to become advocates for the rights of others.

Another reason for the success of the advocacy campaigns was the regular training provided to project staff members to ensure that the basic themes and issues were fully understood and that the campaigns could be executed effectively. In addition, holding regular steering committee meetings to review results and adapt advocacy campaigns and messages as needed was important.

To ensure press coverage of the advocacy campaigns, the project staff informed the media prior to the events and regularly updated the media on the campaign outcomes. In addition, project staff members were well prepared to engage the media in interviews and public forums. These efforts ensured that the issue of HIV-related stigma and discrimination received wider publicity and visibility and strengthened the capacity of women in sex work to speak out openly and advocate for their rights.

Challenges and unforeseen outcomes: Engaging doctors and police in formal training sessions was difficult because of the nature of their work. Therefore, project staff members developed an innovative informal approach to reaching these key stakeholders. The project team also found that morality-related stigma and discrimination require different approaches and take more time to change than stigma that stems from lack of knowledge and fear of transmission. Last, the project team found that the media's understanding of stigma and discrimination was limited, which influenced how sex workers and sex workers living with HIV were portrayed in the media. Specific advocacy efforts targeting the media were developed to address this challenge.

Additional Information

Program references, media coverage, and materials developed:

- A pictorial community monitoring tool on stigma assessment
- More than 20 articles published in many Kannada and English newspapers
- A local TV channel telecast of a program on HIV and women in sex work

Contact information: Pushpa Latha. R, sms-pragati@airtelmail.in

Additional funding, replication, or scale-up opportunities or new partnerships resulting from the project: Prior to the project, the three support organizations for women in sex work were working separately in different areas of Bangalore. Because of the collective recognition among these organizations of the need to foster a more supportive environment for women in sex work, these organizations joined, with support from the NGO Swasti, to write the proposal for SARDM. The resulting partnership between the four organizations proved crucial for implementing and monitoring a large and multifaceted campaign. The success of this partnership demonstrates the value in fostering partnerships between community-based organizations and technical NGOs for the design and implementation of stigma reduction efforts. Additionally, as a direct result of this project, the three support organizations have now launched the Network for Women's Equity and Equality, which they hope will become a regional or national umbrella organization for sex worker support organizations throughout the country.

The Communication Hub

Project title: Celebrating Those Who Care: A Radio Program by Positive Journalists

Implementing organizations: The Communication Hub (TCH), Network of Maharashtra People with HIV (NMP+)

Location: Maharashtra: Konkan, Khandesh, Western Maharashtra, Vidharbha, Marathwada

Background

Program goals: To develop a 13-part radio serial to highlight the stories of people living with HIV and a significant supportive person in their life. By showcasing individuals from all walks of life who support people living with HIV, the project hoped to communicate to the radio listeners what nonstigmatizing and nondiscriminatory behavior is and aimed to inspire audiences to emulate such behavior. A secondary goal was to train people living with HIV in radio journalism so that they could, by participating in this project, attain confidence in using the power of the media to shape public opinion on HIV.

Target audiences: General population and people living with HIV

Primary approach: Media (radio)

Description of intervention: A project partnership was created between TCH and NMP+, and a memorandum of understanding was developed to outline roles and responsibilities of the project team.

With the rural population of Maharashtra as the target, the project team opted to use radio for several reasons. Radio is relatively low cost and reaches a large audience that may not have access to electricity or television, may be mobile, or may have low literacy. All India Radio has near universal reach in Maharashtra, unlike private radio channels that are limited to more urban areas. All India Radio's 20 stations in Maharashtra reach a population of approximately 96.9 million, including about 55.8 million people residing in rural areas.

The start-up process for the radio serial involved meetings with stakeholders such as All India Radio, the selection of people living with HIV to serve as radio journalists, and training. Those selected as radio journalists participated in a three-day training on equipment use, interviewing techniques, and communication skills. During this time, the team conducted a workshop to jointly identify with NMP+ priority themes and issues to be covered in the serial. These discussions led to a design document outlining key content and messages, which served as an essential reference guide in the field for the radio journalists and the scriptwriter.

In addition, as part of the training workshop, the team held a brainstorming session on harmful words that are frequently used in the media and in daily discourse. The team identified better alternatives and came to agreement on guidelines for ensuring that stigmatizing language was not used during the interviews. Consent protocols were also arrived at, and consent forms were designed.

After developing the initial four episodes, the team conducted testing to get audience feedback on the stories. This input informed the development of the remaining episodes. The pretest revealed that the audience was as interested in hearing the voice of people living with HIV as it was in learning about the persons who provided the support. Subsequent episodes featured more stories from people living with HIV, who were seen as the real heroes of the episodes. In the end, the 13-part radio serial weaves stories with critical information on HIV and AIDS. The serial addresses misconceptions about HIV and people living with HIV and provides a means for members of the radio audience to act on what they have heard. Episodes include information on available testing, care and treatment services, and ways to contact NMP+.

To date, the radio serial has not yet been broadcast. The NACO-supported the Maharashtra State AIDS Control Society has recently included the program in its next financial year media budget (April 2010–March 2011), so the project team anticipates the serial will be broadcast over the next year.

Implementation, Results, and Challenges

Measurement strategies: A pretest of four episodes was conducted, and four focus group discussions were held, each with 10–12 participants. Six in-depth interviews with particular members of the community were also completed. A pre- and posttraining survey was conducted with 10 journalists.

Results, key findings, and lessons: All case study respondents, including radio journalists, those interviewed by the radio journalists, and TCH team members talked about their own learning and growth through participation in this project. Those living with HIV trained to be radio journalists discussed the technical skills they learned (for example, using computers and digital recorders). They also gained skills in public speaking and in articulating questions and delivering messages.

The radio journalists felt the interviews were often cathartic and made interviewees proud that their story was important enough to be on radio. Interviewees were glad that their story would benefit others.

The radio journalists greatly appreciated the initial training (three days). However, all agreed that if they had the opportunity to do it over, the initial training would be much longer. In addition, they would add on-the-ground mentoring on recording techniques (for example, how to minimize ambient noise); interviewing techniques (for example, how to ask shorter and sharper questions); and refresher training after a few initial interviews.

Central to the success of project implementation has been the partnership between TCH and NMP+. Both parties described the importance of this partnership and the benefits, learning, and inspiration it brought to each of them. The project also strengthened their understanding of how to forge a productive partnership. The memorandum of understanding signed at the start of the project played a key role in the success of the partnership. Jointly created by the two organizations, it clearly laid out expectations, roles, and responsibilities.

Challenges and unforeseen outcomes: Positive role models were often reluctant to be interviewed for fear of what might happen when the story was broadcast. Because it was important to respond to this challenge within the production time frame, a few studio interviews with experts were conducted to allow the project to address the identified need for more factual information on HIV.

One theme that could not be covered was the workplace setting. The project team found employers reluctant to discuss programs and policies they had put in place for HIV-positive staff, fearing they would send a signal to the public that their organization employed many HIV-positive people, which might result in negative fallout on their corporate image as well as the sale of their products.

Additional Information
Program references, media coverage, and materials developed:

- Process document
- Design document, which was produced with people living with HIV and highlights key messages on stigma and discrimination that should be used in radio
- 13 episodes of a radio serial
- Media coverage of design workshop
- Report of the pretest

Contact information: Sonalini Mirchandani, sonalini@thecommunication hub.com

Additional funding, replication, or scale-up opportunities or new partnerships resulting from the project: The NACO-supported Maharashtra State AIDS

Control Society has recently included the program in its next financial year media budget (April 2010–March 2011). The network has suggested that this experience could be replicated in other states in India, and a similar collaboration involving Indian Network for People Living with HIV/AIDS could be undertaken so that such a program could be made in other languages.

Voluntary Health Association of Tripura

Project title: Integrated Communication Strategy for Tackling HIV and AIDS Stigma and Discrimination in Tripura

Implementing organizations: Voluntary Health Association of Tripura (VHAT) and partner organizations: Pushparaj Club, Yatiya Yuba Sangstha, Vidyasagar Samaj Kalyan Samsad, Ramnagar Mahila Samity, Organization for Rural Survival

Location: Agartala, Tripura state

Background

Program goal: To create general awareness in Agartala about the reduction of stigma by training media personnel and producing and disseminating stigma reduction messages in print and electronic media

Target audiences: Religious leaders, panchayat members, media personnel, members of the defense force (Border Security Force), general community, people living with HIV

Primary approaches: Training, IEC, media coverage

Description of intervention: The VHAT and its partners implemented a range of project activities in the city of Agartala in Tripura state. Project activities included training selected groups on HIV-related stigma and discrimination, holding workshops for journalists in print and electronic media, and providing social and legal support in cases of stigma and discrimination.

Three-day trainings for the religious leaders, panchayat members, media personnel, and members of the Border Security Force (BSF) had approximately 30 participants per training. Media personnel were trained in one-day workshops.

In addition to training, the project aimed to provide social and legal support to people living with HIV affected by stigma and discrimination. At project inception, a brief survey was implemented with the help of partner organizations to identify cases of stigma and discrimination in

Agartala. In the course of the project, 10 cases of stigma and discrimination were documented. The VHAT provided social support to the cases of stigma it came across through community meetings and mobilization. In terms of social support for sex workers, the VHAT organized meetings with community leaders and panchayat members on each case and also discussed HIV prevention with sex workers and arranged regular health checkups for them to facilitate treatment for STIs and ART, if needed. For the children of HIV-positive parents, VHAT members discussed with the parents of other children in the school and community myths surrounding casual transmission of HIV. They emphasized the right to education and participation for all children. In terms of social support for MSM, the project arranged treatment and counseling for those who experienced stigma. The VHAT also provided legal support in one case of discrimination.

Implementation, Results, and Challenges

Measurement strategy: Training and workshop participants completed a pre- and postintervention written evaluation covering the following topics:

- HIV prevention
- STIs
- Use of condoms and debunking myths surrounding condoms
- Referrals to Integrated Counseling and Testing Centers in government hospitals
- ART and services available for STIs
- Harmful effects of stigma and discrimination
- Benefits of reducing stigma
- Information about social and legal support systems.

Results, key findings, and lessons: The written evaluation indicated a 60 percentage point increase, on average, in knowledge among respondents.

Within the 18 months of the project period, training was provided to 247 religious leaders, 231 panchayat members, and 105 BSF members.

In all, the project trained 62 media personnel in one-day media workshops. As a result, in the first phase of the project, key messages were developed through detailed discussions with local media personnel and International Center for Research on Women staff members, and 500 posters and 2,000 stickers were printed and disseminated. In the second phase of the project, 500 copies of a booklet on HIV and other STIs were printed and distributed. Additionally, stigma reduction messages were displayed on billboards at 10 major intersections in the city.

As a result of the training, panchayat members organized meetings to promote stigma reduction and are now more cooperative and involved with HIV initiatives. Several religious leaders who participated in the training continue to disseminate messages about stigma to their followers, to disseminate condoms among vulnerable groups, to refer on average three or four persons per week for testing, and to assist with vulnerable groups in the testing camps. Trained members of the BSF are now motivated to help refer people living with HIV to an antiretroviral center in Agartala.

Challenges and unforeseen outcomes: The VHAT faced some challenges because religious leaders initially tended to be reluctant to attend training on HIV. The majority of the religious leaders trained were Christian (of 44 mosques, only three sent imams, and only Hindu temples that traditionally have a social wing sent a priest for training). Discussing MSM with religious leaders during the training was also challenging because it is a culturally taboo subject. The VHAT appealed to the faith leaders for their help in a nonthreatening and nonjudgmental way. Through sharing the real-life stories and case studies and through group discussions, the VHAT gradually opened up the discussions about MSM. Religious leaders who attended the first training later worked as motivators for subsequent groups of religious leaders.

Additional Information

Program references, media coverage, and materials developed: Many VHAT activities were published in local newspapers and broadcast from local radio and television channels. Project activities generated more than 50 news stories on HIV and AIDS, which ran on media outlets, including All India Radio, Doordarshan Kendra Agartala, Akash Tripura, and NE TV.

The news and articles covered issues related to workshops on reduction of stigma and discrimination organized by the VHAT and its partners throughout the state, the importance of awareness for reduction of stigma and discrimination, life stages of transgender groups, establishment of a community care center and other available services in Agartala, and basic information regarding HIV and AIDS.

The following newspapers published articles on HIV-related stigma and discrimination reduction and other relevant issues during the project period: *Syandan Patrika, Daily Deshar Katha, Tripura Times, Tripura Darpan, Tripura Prabaha, Dainik Sambad, Ajker Fariad, Tripura Observer, and Uttarer Jana Barta.*

Contact information: Sreelekha Ray, vha_tripura@rediffmail.com

Additional funding, replication, or scale-up opportunities or new partnerships resulting from the project: The VHAT started working with female sex workers and MSM with support from the Tripura State AIDS Control Society and the Department of Health and Family Welfare.

We Care Social Service Society

Project title: Promotion of Community Discussion and Debate Using Traditional Folk Media Known as *Therukoothu* (Street Drama)

Implementing organization: We Care Social Service Society

Location: 10 villages of Kancheepuram district, Tamil Nadu (Aakkur, Anumanthai, Katchipattu, Mamandur, Nerumpur, Padalam, Padappai, Singaperumal Koil, Thiruvanthavar, and Vandalur)

Background

Program goals: To use a traditional Tamilian street drama (*therukoothu*) to educate and promote discussion about HIV and its associated stigma and discrimination

Target audiences: People living with HIV, general public

Primary approach: Traditional theater

Description of intervention: A professional scriptwriter developed an initial storyline, and the HIV and stigma themes were added through a script development workshop that included people living with HIV, HIV experts, troupe members, and theater professionals. In the workshop, the team drew on data from interviews with people living with HIV from three networks in the district. The script combined well-known traditional, mythical stories with real-life experiences of people living with HIV, moving between the two and drawing parallels between modern life with HIV and the ancient stories. A narrator (*kattiakkaran*) weaves the past and present storylines together. The script continued to evolve throughout the training process and performances, integrating new ideas brought forward by the theater troupe as the process of performing unfolded and taking into account audience questions and reactions.

Although the original idea had been that the troupe would consist only of people living with HIV (nonprofessional actors), the impracticality of this idea quickly became apparent. Therefore, the project formed a mixed troupe of nonprofessional actors living with HIV and professional actors, which ended up providing unique opportunities for stigma reduction among the HIV-negative performers. The performance team consisted of seven professional theater performers, five nonprofessional performers living with HIV, and three HIV-negative volunteers. The project trained the performers for two months on an array of issues including self-esteem, group dynamics, team building, life skills, self-presentation in the villages, script development, and *therukoothu*-style performance.

With the help of the Tamil Nadu Network of Positive People, the project team identified 10 villages where at least four people living with HIV resided and where stigma was particularly problematic. Key leaders in each of these villages, including leaders from youth and women's groups, were contacted and invited to form the project support committees. These committees took full ownership of the program. At their own expense, they organized boarding and lodging for the troupe, arranged a sound system for the performance, and generated publicity about the event in the community.

The troupe performed the play for three consecutive nights in 10 villages in Kancheepuram district. The play stopped at various points for discussion and information exchange with audience members. The troupe encouraged audience members to ask questions, offering prizes for participation. The troupe stayed in the village for four days, thus allowing performers opportunities to interact with village members and provide information about and referrals for voluntary counseling and testing and care services.

Implementation, Results, and Challenges

Measurement strategies: Twenty focus group discussions and 64 key informant interviews were conducted with women, self-help groups, youth, village leaders, and village elders.

Results, key findings, and lessons: Five people living with HIV were trained to perform and participate in community theater and discussions.

Three performances were held in each of 10 villages.

Audience participation increased over time, and people living with HIV in the villages where performances were held came forward to access services available from NGOs and government hospitals.

Knowing some of the actors were living with HIV had a powerful effect on audiences, intensifying the messages delivered during performances. After seeing the play, villagers talked about how they had not realized the harm done by stigma and discrimination and how, now that they understood, they would change their behavior. They also talked at length about the importance of supporting people living with HIV in their efforts to lead a healthy and productive life.

A key to success was creating ownership among people in the villages. In each village, volunteers served on village committees to raise funds to house and feed the theater troupe for three nights, procured equipment and space, printed flyers, and generated publicity for the show. The presence of the theater troupe in the village was also important. Villagers conversed with troupe members during the day, asking questions and in some cases seeking care and service referrals. These interactions also allowed the troupe to alter the performance to respond to specific questions raised during the day.

Challenges and unforeseen outcomes: Discussion of HIV-related issues met a lot of resistance in the rural community. Successful implementation required patience and persistence to convince village gatekeepers to allow the play in their locale. Leaders in many villages were initially hesitant because of the topic. However, once a few performances had been held and word spread about how good the play was, villages began calling up to ask for performances. Another challenge was striking the right balance between entertainment to hold the audience's attention and delivering informational messages. The script continually evolved, sharpened through repeated performances and audience feedback.

Additional Information
Program references, media coverage, and materials developed:

- Training curriculum for training of troupe members in *therukoothu*
- Three scripts for *therukoothu*
- Video documentation
- Publication of process report

Contact information: A. Antony Samy, wecareindia@gmail.com

Additional funding, replication, or scale-up opportunities or new partnerships resulting from the project: Even after the project ended, demand for the play has continued to grow. Other villages have been calling to request performances; two local corporations have sponsored performances in additional villages (beyond what was possible in the SARDM budget); and the United Nations Children's Fund has asked We Care to submit a proposal to conduct the play in more villages.

CHAPTER 15

Nepal

Federation of Sexual and Gender Minorities Nepal

Project title: Beauty and Brains in Action to Tackle HIV/AIDS Stigma and Discrimination

Implementing organizations: Federation of Sexual and Gender Minorities Nepal (FSGMN) and partner organizations: Blue Diamond Society (BDS), Kathmandu; Naulo Bihani-Pokhara, Western Region; Human Conscious Society, Narayangadh, Central Region; BDS Biratnagar, Biratnagar, Eastern Region; BDS Dhangadi, Dhangadi, Far Western Region; Western Star Nepalgunj, Nepalgunj, Midwestern Region

Location: Five regions in Nepal (Narayangadh, Central; Pokhara, Western; Biratnagar, Eastern; Dhangadi, Far Western; Nepalgunj, Midwestern)

Background

Program goals: To empower men who have sex with men (MSM) and transgender communities and to educate the general population and service providers by giving visibility to MSM and transgender individuals, giving them the opportunity to show that they are part of society, highlighting the misconceptions that fuel stigma and discrimination, and enabling MSM and transgender individuals to make their own recommendations on reducing stigma and discrimination through a series of beauty pageants for MSM and transgender individuals, with the winners taking on roles as ambassadors for the community

Target audiences: General population, MSM and transgender communities

Primary approaches: Beauty pageant and ambassadorship of winners

Description of intervention: The intervention consisted of five regional beauty pageants and one national pageant to identify national and regional ambassadors among the MSM and transgender communities. Sixty-one pageant contestants received five days of preparatory training, including sessions about public speaking, choreography, and interpersonal communication skills; HIV and other sexually transmitted infections; and human rights and stigma and discrimination. Through songs, dance, drama, poems, and other performances, pageant contestants went on to deliver messages about HIV prevention and other issues faced by the transgender community during the competition. Winners were selected on the basis of level of confidence exhibited, presentation, personality, and subject matter delivered. The top three contestants from each region advanced to the national competition, where the national and regional ambassadors were selected.

Five regional winners were declared and appointed as regional HIV ambassadors, and one contestant was selected as the national ambassador. The appointed ambassadors were then formally supported by FSGMN to help lead a public advocacy campaign, a media campaign, and a political and constitutional rights campaign in their localities. This support included additional training to increase knowledge of HIV and AIDS–related stigma, voluntary counseling and testing, advocacy skills, media campaigning skills, and reporting skills on human rights violations. The training was supported by funds from the United Nations Development Programme and BDS. The objective of the campaigns was to promote the health and human rights of the transgender community by coordinating with local civil society organizations, human rights organizations, media houses, and organizations working on HIV and AIDS. Throughout the project, ambassadors participated in public forums, talk programs, seminars, and other gatherings to rally people around lesbian, gay, bisexual, transgender, and intersex (LGBTI) issues and to support their human rights.

Implementation, Results, and Challenges
Measurement strategies:

- Process and monitoring data
- Media coverage

- End of project workshop with ambassadors to document their experience of participation
- Legislative, local government, and other action taken as a result of the advocacy campaign

Results, key findings, and lessons: The reach of the project was broad. While 1,500 individuals attended the six pageants, the indirect audience was estimated to be quite large because the events were subsequently highlighted on television (TV) and in print media. The HIV ambassadors went on to lead or participate in 228 advocacy events throughout the country during the project period. These advocacy campaigns resulted in a number of positive outcomes. Foremost among them were the following:

- Expanded coverage of LBGTI issues in the print, TV, and electronic media, including the establishment of a weekly, 30-minute *Third Sex* program on the national TV station dedicated to promoting LBGTI human rights, which has been airing every Saturday since August 2009
- Inclusion of LBGTI human rights in political party manifestos and constitutional concept notes, which led to the inclusion of text regarding the problem of identity and protective provisions for LBGTI individuals in preliminary drafts of the new constitution
- First-time allocation by the Nepalese government of more than NrP 3 million in the fiscal year 2009/10 budget for the promotion of LBGTI human rights
- Expanded interest in LBGTI issues among researchers, students, activists, national and international journalists, publications, and Web-hosting organizations
- Boosted self-esteem, increased knowledge of HIV, more acceptance from families, and less teasing and harassment from the public reported by the HIV ambassadors themselves.

The success of this intervention was owed in large part to the strong relationships that FSGMN built with key stakeholders, including government officials, at the beginning of the project and consistent engagement with these stakeholders throughout project implementation.

Challenges and unforeseen outcomes: The frequently postponed and then canceled Miss Nepal 2008 pageant and the debates surrounding it were an unforeseen event that helped increase public attention to the similar Beauty and Brains events. One challenge faced was the limited funds available for the ambassadors to organize events following the pageants. Instead, they demonstrated their activism by participating in events to which they were invited.

Additional Information

Program references, media coverage, and materials developed: A DVD (digital video disc) was produced of all six events organized in different parts of Nepal, including the training period and interviews with the participants before and after the training and events describing the changes in their capacity, perceptions, and confidence level.

Project glimpses and articles can be found on the following Web sites:

- "Gay Beauty Pageant Defies Maoists," http://timesofindia.indiatimes .com/Gay_beauty_pageant_defies_Maoists/articleshow/2014387.cms
- "Miss Nepal Derailed but Miss Gay Right on Course," http://www .dnaindia.com/report.asp?newsid=1213835,
  http://www.thaindian.com/newsportal/world-news/miss-nepal-derailed-but-miss-gay-right-on-course-with-image_100130752.html,
  http://beacononline.wordpress.com/2008/12/16/
- "Miss Beauty and Brain," http://www.sarasansar.com/event/miss_beauty _n_brain/
- "Nepali Transwoman Eager for Miss International Queen Challenge," http://transgriot.blogspot.com/search/label/pageants
- "Miss World Transsexual—International Queen," http://miss-interna tionalqueen.blogspot.com/2009/11/miss-nepal-sandhya-lama.html
- "Asia Celebrity News," http://entertainment.sg.msn.com/photos/ photos.aspx?cp-documentid=3682484&page=18
- "News from Nepal," http://actionbeautyandbrains.wordpress.com/
- "Nepali TG Beauty Queens on Front Page of the Prestigious Magazine *VOW* Nepal," http://lgbtbangladesh.wordpress.com/2009/05/07/ nepali-tg-beauty-queens-on-front-page-of-the-prestigious-magazine-vow-nepal/
- *VOW* magazine, http://www.vownepal.com/
- "Miss Gay Nepal Now Eyes the World," http://blog.taragana.com/law/ 2009/09/27/miss-gay-nepal-now-eyes-the-world-13191/, http://www.mynews.in/News/Miss_Gay_Nepal_now_eyes_the_world_ N26743.html#
- "Beauty and Brains (in Post Production)," http://www.eggplant12.co. uk/news.php?action=displayItem&id=16
- *Weekly Nepal* magazine, http://www.weeklynepal.com/newsite2/ component/publication/?task=display&view=current&pub_id=35

- "Pastors' Seminar on Bible and Homosexuality—with Featured Talks from Gay Nepali Christians," http://www.othersheepexecsite.com/Asia_2009_Nepal_Other_Sheep_July_5_Seminar_for_area_pastors_Kathmandu_Nepal_Parelli_Ortiz.html
- "Miss Gay Nepal," http://www.criticalbeauty.com/Journal_Dec_2008.html.

Contact information: Sunil Babu Pant, beauty.and.brain2008@gmail.com; Subash Pokharel, bluediamondsociety@yahoo.com

Additional funding, replication, or scale-up opportunities or new partnerships resulting from the project: The ambassadors, along with other participants through their campaigns, convinced Save the Children USA, the Family Planning Association, and the Global Fund to Fight AIDS, Tuberculosis, and Malaria to bring prevention programs on HIV for MSM and transgender communities to 14 districts in Nepal. FSGMN is now implementing the HIV prevention program targeting MSM and transgender communities in 14 districts, employing 200 MSM and transgender community members. Four regional ambassadors were promoted to this project and are now taking responsibility for organizing district-level prevention programs. FSGMN is also engaging in frequent meetings with interested donors to seek opportunities to expand its stigma reduction efforts. The BDS at the South Asian–level received support from the Global Fund to Fight AIDS, Tuberculosis, and Malaria for five years, from 2012 to 2017, but the amount for Nepal is not yet finalized.

Himalayan Association against STI-AIDS

Project title: Addressing HIV and AIDS Related Stigma and Discrimination through Social, Economic, and Institutional Interventions in Achham District

Implementing organizations: Himalayan Association against STI-AIDS (HASTI-AIDS) and New Diyalo Samaj (Achham)

Location: Achham district, Seti Zone, Far Western Region, Nepal

Background
Program goals: To reduce the occurrence and effects of HIV-related stigma and discrimination among the people of the Achham district in the Far Western Region of Nepal

Target audiences: General population, people living with HIV, migrants and their families, health workers, teachers, students, journalists, volunteers, opinion leaders

Primary approaches: Training, outreach activities

Description of intervention: The project sought to build partnerships and strengthen capacity for local government and nongovernmental organizations (NGOs) to participate in HIV stigma reduction efforts. To achieve this goal, HASTI-AIDS facilitated an HIV stigma reduction workshop with 36 people from the District AIDS Coordination Committee (DACC). This workshop aimed to enhance collaboration among government stakeholders at the local level and to help institutionalize stigma reduction efforts to ensure the sustainability of their efforts.

HASTI-AIDS also facilitated two sensitization workshops attended by 63 teachers, students, health service providers, and other "gatekeepers" in the community. The workshops, which sought to strengthen the capacity of key stakeholders in the community to participate in stigma reduction activities, provided an overview of HIV and stigma and discrimination, a picture of HIV, and the effects of stigma in Achham. Activities were included to promote brainstorming around ideas for stigma reduction in the district.

Strengthening the support system for people living with HIV was another key objective of the project. To accomplish this goal, HASTI-AIDS trained 37 peer educators and female community health volunteers in stigma reduction. The peer educators and community health volunteers subsequently conducted outreach and counseling for people living with HIV and affected families through household visits in eight villages: Basti, Jalpadevi, Kuntibandali, Mangalsen, Mastamandu, Nauthana, Ridikot, and Siddeshor. Each peer educator visited approximately 60 households per month for six months (June–November 2009). In addition, peer educators conducted outreach with migrants and their families using a combination of education and counseling on HIV, sexually transmitted infections (STIs), and HIV-related stigma and discrimination; distribution of condoms and information, education, and communication materials; and referrals for STI treatment, voluntary counseling and testing, and antiretroviral therapy.

Two additional salient activities supported by the project were street dramas and an ongoing radio program. The selected local street drama group performed during local festivals at nine different locations in Achham. The radio program, airing on a popular local FM station known to the community, broadcast an ongoing radio drama and expert views. HASTI-AIDS participated in monthly meetings to discuss the content for the radio programs and was able to promote the inclusion of stigma reduction messages in the radio shows.

Implementation, Results, and Challenges

Measurement strategies:

- Ten focus group discussions with migrants and their spouses, teachers and students, people living with HIV, and health service providers were conducted to assess the level of knowledge about HIV in general and related stigma and discrimination in particular.
- Brief, pre- and posttraining surveys were conducted with people living with HIV and prospective group facilitators.
- Three review meetings with peer educators were conducted to assess how the knowledge and skills learned during the training were disseminated during home visits and contacts with community members.
- Five review meetings were conducted with people living with HIV groups to assess progress on stigma reduction.
- Process indicators were used.

Results, key findings, and lessons: The project activities resulted in a number of important outcomes. First, as a result of the DACC workshop, stigma reduction has become a priority on the DACC's agenda, and the people living with HIV support group is now invited as a permanent observer to DACC meetings.

On the basis of its past experience, HASTI-AIDS decided to emphasize interpersonal communication rather than group education for the outreach activities. The project staff reported that this more personalized approach led to reductions in the incidents of discrimination toward people living with HIV. For example, people living with HIV made fewer reports of being prevented from using public taps, from sharing food with their families at home, and from participating in social events. Also, a large increase has occurred in the number of clients coming for voluntary counseling and testing since the outreach efforts began.

Peer educators who participated in the review meetings indicated that overall stigma and discrimination in the community are decreasing. The migrants have started taking the initiative to communicate with peers in Mumbai, and the wives of migrants have started taking the initiative to keep condoms at home because of the counseling they received during home visits by peer educators. Peer educators also noted that the capacity of housewives to negotiate condom usage when their husbands return home seems to have improved. In addition, school dropouts appear to have decreased substantially, especially for children in grades 8 through 10, which indicates a drop in the trend of going to Mumbai among this age group.

As a result of the project, members of the support group for people living with HIV started crisis counseling, which resulted in increased numbers of people living with HIV seeking care at health facilities. People living with HIV participating in the project also noted that community home-based care through such support groups is more effective than conventional institution-based care, especially in the remote hills in Nepal.

The street drama performances and the ongoing radio program proved to be effective channels for increasing understanding of HIV-related stigma in the community.

Challenges and unforeseen outcomes: The remote location of the intervention areas and prolonged disruption of road transport caused an initial delay in the implementation of programs. Identifying a person with the technical capacity to properly monitor and evaluate the project activities was also a challenge.

Additional Information
Program references, media coverage, and materials developed:

- News on the training program, sensitization workshop, DACC workshop, focus group discussions, and street drama were aired by local Rama Roshan FM radio station and local papers.
- The inaugural program was attended by public figures such as Constituent Assembly members, local political personalities, the chief district officer, the local development officer, the district police chief, the chief of the District Health Office, and journalists.

Contact information: Nirmal Kumar Bista, President, hastiaids@mcmail .com.np; nkbista@yahoo.com

Additional funding, replication, or scale-up opportunities or new partnerships resulting from the project: Because this project was the first in the district to work on stigma and discrimination, a general level of awareness has been created for including this important issue in HIV-related work. Some groups have included stigma and discrimination in their ongoing programs, and others have indicated that they will do so in the future.

Currently, no explicit intent has been shown by the government or donors to work with HASTI-AIDS in this area. HASTI-AIDS is currently seeking additional funds to scale up its stigma reduction efforts.

National NGOs Network Group against AIDS–Nepal

Project title: Creating PLHA-Friendly Hospitals: Improving the Hospital Environment for HIV-Positive Clients in Nepalese Regional Hospitals

Implementing organizations: National NGOs Network Group against AIDS–Nepal (Nangan)

Location: Teku, Kathmandu; Pokhara, Kaski; Nepalgunj, Banke

Background

Program goals: To improve the hospital environment for HIV-positive clients in Nepalese regional hospitals

Target audiences: Health workers in three government hospitals, HIV-positive patients accessing care at the three study hospitals

Primary approaches: Training-of-trainers (TOT) and information, education, and communication materials on stigma and discrimination

Description of intervention: The intervention used a TOT model supported by a client satisfaction committee. A working task team provided guidance on project activities. Health care providers, people living with HIV, and government health officials were extensively involved in establishing a quality assurance system for government hospitals. The project organized a review of existing practices of HIV and AIDS–related treatment and care and developed a hospital checklist. Nangan activists were placed in each hospital. Because Nangan is a network of NGOs, it has health activist volunteers in all regions. Their responsibilities are to work on behalf of Nangan in the region, disseminate important messages to the networked NGOs, keep a close eye on the families of people living with HIV and the hospital, organize network meetings to support people living with HIV, and create a friendly environment for them at home and in the hospital.

Implementation, Results, and Challenges

Measurement strategies: A 10-question client satisfaction survey (of 204 people) was implemented in each hospital at three points during November and June 2009 (baseline, midline, and end line) to determine the level of client satisfaction with hospital services. These surveys were conducted by volunteers three times in each hospital, and nine sets of data were collected. Client exit interviews were done in the hospital setting where antiretroviral medicines are dispensed.

Four monitoring visits were conducted throughout the project using pre- and postintervention direct observation.

Results, key findings, and lessons: The project conducted an initial TOT program with 66 health workers (who were selected by senior management) across the three hospitals. Each hospital then formed a core group of trainers (health workers who participated in the TOT program) to plan, prepare, and implement training for an additional 399 staff members. A client satisfaction committee, consisting of staff and client representatives, was formed to support the project team at the hospital level. Training reports were shared with the client satisfaction committee at monthly meetings in each hospital. At the project level, a working task team provided guidance and suggestions for project activities.

All 339 staff members at the three hospitals were trained: Sukra Raj Tropical (122), Western Regional (132), and Bheri Zonal (85).

A review of existing policies and practices regarding HIV and AIDS–related treatment and care and a series of consultative meetings with the working task team and policy makers informed the development of a hospital checklist, "Friendly Hospital Checklist for Individuals Living with HIV and AIDS." The checklist is aligned with international and national HIV and AIDS and human rights declarations for people living with HIV. It was endorsed by National Centre for AIDS and STI Control and the Ministry of Health and Population.

The project collected 204 client satisfaction surveys from June to November 2009. The survey results, which showed positive changes in client satisfaction over time, were compiled and shared with the three participating hospitals.

One-day regional workshops were held in each of the hospitals from October to December 2009. Regional workshops focused on sharing information about Nangan's activities thus far and the results of the South Asia Region Development Marketplace project. Hospital workers, NGO staff members, and some people living with HIV (unidentified) were present in the workshop. In each workshop, updates—including the results of the client satisfaction survey—were presented to the hospital employees and client satisfaction committee members. The service providers were keenly interested in knowing the results of the client satisfaction survey.

Sagarmatha Television produced and broadcast a documentary of Nangan's work, including activities such as the Creating PLHA-Friendly Hospitals project as part of the Health Is Wealth program.

The client exit survey revealed the project's success in the following areas: increased knowledge about safe and friendly practices, improved communication among staff members, increased capacity to apply safety measures, and improved client satisfaction regarding decreasing stigma and discrimination against people living with HIV from service providers.

Challenges and unforeseen outcomes: Nangan had ambitious objectives to carry out in a short span of time, with little time for sharing of its achievements. The project will achieve greater influence if the successes, including the monitoring results, are shared more widely, and can serve as model for replication among other health facilities. Frequent strikes delayed activities.

Additional Information

Program references, media coverage, and materials developed: Brochure focusing on stigma and discrimination and the concept of a friendly hospital for people living with AIDS

Contact information: Usha Jha, ushajha05@yahoo.com

Additional funding, replication, or scale-up opportunities or new partnerships resulting from the project: The political situation in Nepal is unstable, but Nangan will continue advocacy efforts with the Ministry of Health and Population to replicate aspects of the project. The minister of health has expressed appreciation of the efforts of various programs.

CHAPTER 16

Pakistan

Integrated Health Services

Project title: Advocacy Campaign to Reduce AIDS Stigma by Creating "HIV Forums" at Colleges in Islamabad

Implementing organization: Integrated Health Services (IHS)

Location: Islamabad

Background

Program goals: To raise awareness among university students about HIV, AIDS, and stigma and discrimination and to work toward promoting stigma reduction in the general community

Target audience: University and college students 17 to 25 years of age

Primary approaches: Organization of HIV youth forums, sensitization and training of youth forum members, community sensitization by youth forum members

Description of intervention: The project team mapped local private colleges and universities in Islamabad that might consider forming HIV youth forums. The team developed an introductory letter including a summary of the project for the director of the Federal Directorate of Education and the secretary of education and met with the two officials to obtain their approval of the project. The team then selected 12 schools that met the following eligibility criteria: (a) the schools served students 17 years of age and older and (b) implementation of a successful program seemed feasible given student interests and strengths. When the final 12 schools were selected, project staff members visited the schools and met with college and university officials. A faculty member or teacher on staff at each school was designated as the HIV youth forum coordinator.

Once the teams had been selected and the coordinator identified, project staff members visited all 12 schools to provide information about the project to deans, principals, and student affairs administrators. Project activities were scheduled at that time in coordination with the school calendar. Such activities included the project staff's presentation on HIV, AIDS, stigma, and discrimination. Visits began in September 2008, and by January 2009, all of the schools had been visited and the first presentation by the project team had been conducted. In mid-January, training of forum participants began. Some delay occurred in scheduling the trainings because of school examination schedules. Student forum members were provided an information booklet and fact sheet about HIV and AIDS as well as handouts, which were distributed during the project staff presentations at each school. Following the training, HIV student forum members created awareness among their peers, friends, families, and community about HIV and AIDS by holding awareness-raising sessions and one-on-one discussions. Forum members also arranged creative activities such as dramas, speech contests, and theater performances on themes related to HIV and stigma in their respective colleges and universities. They also performed voluntary activities providing counseling to people living with HIV and their families.

Implementation, Results, and Challenges
Measurement strategies:

- Pre- and postintervention surveys were conducted among a random sample of students at five Islamabad colleges and universities. The survey assessed knowledge and attitudes regarding HIV and AIDS, level of awareness of stigma and what it means, and attitudes of students toward people living with HIV and AIDS. Students provided informed consent before participating in the surveys. In total, 462 students were surveyed at baseline and 445 were surveyed following the intervention.
- Monthly report forms were completed by HIV youth forum coordinators.
- Registration forms were completed.

Results, key findings, and lessons: Overall, 1,674 students attended the HIV-awareness presentations, of whom 362 became members of the HIV student forums at the 12 universities. By the end of the project, more students had joined, for a total of 443 youth forum members. Eleven students participated in individual counseling sessions with people living with HIV. In addition to holding monthly awareness sessions, all 12 forums engaged in other activities related to HIV themes, such as speech competitions, dramas, and theatrical performances. The 12 forums held a total of 13 such events. The key lesson learned was that youth in Pakistan are an appropriate audience for reproductive health education, including awareness about HIV and stigma, and can be actively involved in community sensitization activities. The tremendous energy of youth and students can be harnessed to increase health awareness by creating and organizing forums, clubs, or societies at colleges and universities.

The evaluation indicated increases in general knowledge about HIV, AIDS, and stigma. In addition, the fear of HIV infection through casual contact with a person living with HIV and the shame and blame directed toward people living with HIV decreased by the end of the project. For example, at baseline, 16 percent of students surveyed stated that they had heard of the word *stigma* compared with 60 percent at end line. Similarly, 84 percent provided a correct definition for HIV at end line, compared with 51 percent at baseline. Knowledge of antiretroviral therapy also increased substantially. Although at baseline 25 percent of students agreed that "people with HIV and AIDS should feel ashamed of themselves," only 9 percent agreed with that statement at end line. In addition, at baseline 32 percent of students were afraid of becoming infected with HIV by sharing plates or utensils with a person living with HIV, compared with 10 percent following the intervention. The percentage of students who reported speaking with their family about HIV and AIDS increased substantially over the course of the project (from 27 percent at baseline to 91 percent at end line), which indicates that increasing awareness of HIV, AIDS, and stigma among students can provide an important entry point for informing families about these critical issues.

Challenges and unforeseen outcomes: Convincing the administrators and students of private colleges and universities to take part in the cause of creating awareness among the community about HIV and AIDS was difficult. This difficulty stemmed from concern that starting HIV youth forums and creating awareness would expose students to sex and reproductive health education, which in Pakistan is still considered something educational institutions should not do. To overcome this challenge, IHS met numerous times with the administrators to convince them that professional educators have a critical role to play in ensuring that students have correct scientific information about sexual health and HIV and are provided with this information in an ethical and truthful manner.

Additional Information
Program references, media coverage, and materials developed:

- "Fast Facts" sheet for members
- Youth forum HIV information booklet

Contact information: Muhammad Asim Mahmood Khan, IHS Pakistan, asim@ihspakistan.com; ihspakistan@hotmail.com

Additional funding, replication, or scale-up opportunities or new partnerships resulting from the project: IHS is currently working to develop a reproductive health syllabus for teachers to enable them to be a continuous and consistent source of reproductive health information for students. Teachers are the main focus of this effort because previous experience has shown that universities and parents are much more supportive if such issues are addressed internally rather than by bringing in outside experts to provide such information. IHS is also planning to educate journalists to highlight the importance of including reproductive health curricula in schools and colleges.

New Light AIDS Control Society

Project title: Reducing Stigma to Improve Uptake for Antiretroviral Treatment and Community Home-Based Care among People Living with HIV and AIDS, Men Who Have Sex with Men, and Individuals from the Transgender Community

Implementing organizations: New Light AIDS Control Society (NLACS)

Location: Karachi, Lahore, and Multan districts

Background
Program goals: To increase access of people living with HIV and men who have sex with men (MSM) to antiretroviral treatment and community home-based care without stigma and discrimination

Target audiences: MSM, people living with HIV, transgender individuals, key stakeholders

Primary approach: Training of trainers

Description of intervention: The project involved training of trainers on HIV, AIDS, and stigma for MSM, individuals from the transgender community, and their friends and relatives. Of the 24 persons trained, 16 went on to become master trainers. The master trainers then trained a total of 390 other MSM and transgender individuals on HIV-related issues in 26 training sessions held during the project period. Master trainers also led seminars for health care providers and media personnel.

The NLACS staff worked to establish or strengthen referral systems and links for treatment and care services for these marginalized groups. The referral systems were strengthened through regular meetings with health care providers. In addition, structured awareness campaigns on HIV and AIDS were organized within the target community. Ten case studies exploring the everyday issues and problems faced by MSM and people living with HIV were prepared and disseminated in Urdu and English among important stakeholders, including MSM and people living with HIV, nongovernmental organizations (NGOs), the general public, and government institutions. Last, English-language classes were offered to interested MSM and transgender individuals as a way to enhance capacity.

Implementation, Results, and Challenges
Measurement strategies:

- Baseline and end-line surveys were conducted to assess the project's effect.
- Pre- and posttraining evaluations were conducted among the master trainers and the additional trainees.
- In-depth interviews were conducted with 26 selected MSM, transgender individuals, and people living with HIV at target locations in Lahore, Multan, and Karachi to develop case studies.
- NLACS completed monthly activity progress reports.

Results, key findings, and lessons: Following the structured awareness-raising campaigns among MSM and transgender communities, 377 individuals visited the NLACS offices for voluntary counseling and testing (VCT). They also received information on HIV and AIDS during counseling sessions. Of those who were tested, 16 were diagnosed as HIV-positive and linked with the home-based care services provided by NLACS. These services included twice-monthly home-based care visits. A total of 64 home visits were conducted, during which 90 family members of the 16 people living with HIV and MSM were sensitized on HIV and AIDS.

In four separate seminars, 46 media personnel and 43 health care workers were provided with basic information about MSM and transgender individuals, such as the distinction between these two groups and the challenges and obstacles they face, including their specific health care needs. These seminars led to enhanced cooperation and support from both the media personnel and the health care workers. For example, media personnel made commitments to reduce stigma and discrimination through more accurate reporting in print and broadcast media and agreed to receive news stories and information from NLACS for dissemination.

Efforts to strengthen ties with local hospitals and VCT centers, both public and private, expanded the NLACS referral system to 36 villages and included the addition of seven hospitals and one VCT center. Building links, promoting VCT, and providing home-based visits all increased identification of those who needed services and ensured links to care and treatment. According to monitoring data, demand for condoms increased dramatically over the project period. A total of 26,746 condoms were distributed in the MSM and transgender communities through awareness-raising campaigns, meetings, and training sessions and during monitoring visits.

Overall, the project raised awareness within the MSM and transgender communities about HIV and AIDS and available treatment and care services. In addition, the project provided space for discussion and reflection through workshops with peer master trainers in each district. Involvement of leaders from the community of MSM in the implementation process promoted interest and meaningful participation and made possible wide dissemination of messages about HIV, stigma, and related issues.

Of trained MSM and transgender individuals, 60 percent reported to the NLACS monitoring team that their attitude had improved and that they had gained the confidence needed to handle situations related to stigma and discrimination from the local community.

Two press conferences, one in Lahore and one in Karachi, were organized by NLACS and Action Aid–Pakistan to discuss MSM and transgender issues. A large number of MSM and transgender individuals participated in these events and confidently expressed their concerns and problems in front of electronic and print media representatives.

Following are some of the basic results from the evaluation data collected among MSM and transgender groups before and after the intervention:

- Initially, the target groups were reluctant to talk about sexually transmitted infections (STIs) and HIV and AIDS issues. However, they gradually gained confidence and were eager to learn about STIs, and they convinced their friends and partners to learn about these issues.
- At baseline, usage of condoms and lubricant was quite low, but almost all respondents reported using condoms consistently at end line.
- At baseline, participants were afraid of being identified as HIV positive, but at end line, respondents not only came for testing, but those who identified as HIV positive also began using antiretroviral treatment services.
- As a result of this intervention, most of the targeted members suggested that such programs should continue because many people still do not have accurate information about HIV and AIDS.
- At baseline, many respondents were reluctant to go to doctors because of the discriminatory attitude toward MSM and transgender individuals. However, at end line, those sensitized are now more willing to take their partners to doctors for VCT and treatment services.

Challenges and unforeseen outcomes: Many of the master trainers had full-time jobs and could not conduct trainings during the day, so training sessions were scheduled on weekends to accommodate trainers with full-time employment. Fluency in English was limited among the MSM and transgender individuals involved in the project. Therefore, the project team translated training material into Urdu for these target groups. The project staff observed that inability to speak and read English posed obstacles for some in accessing care and in gaining permanent employment. Although the project offered an English certificate course, only five participants enrolled and received certificates. The project staff decided to continue this component despite low uptake.

Initially, people living with HIV hesitated to share their problems with the staff, but after the sensitization and home-based care visits, they now have the confidence to talk about problems they are facing.

Additional Information

Program references, media coverage, and materials developed:

- Four-day training manual for MSM master trainers on HIV and STIs
- The training manual *Dost se Dost ko Taleem* (*Education from One Friend to Another*)
- Media coverage on World AIDS Day when the "Silent Words" case study was launched

Contact information: Asher Bhatti, newlightaids@gmail.com

Additional funding, replication, or scale-up opportunities or new partnerships resulting from the project: In Karachi, MSM and transgender individuals formed a group called Participatory Organisation for Empowerment of Transgender (POET) to advocate and inform the government and local community on the rights of MSM and transgender individuals.

NLACS is currently seeking support from the U.S. Agency for International Development and others to continue and scale up the project activities piloted.

Pakistan Press Foundation

Project title: Capacity Development of Media and Civil Society Organizations to Improve Coverage of HIV/AIDS

Implementing organization: Pakistan Press Foundation (PPF)

Location: Abbottabad, Karachi, Lahore, Multan, Nathia Gali, Quetta, and Sukkur

Background

Program goals: To reduce stigma and discrimination against HIV in Pakistan (and Pakistan-administered Kashmir) society through capacity development of the media and civil society organizations (CSOs), leading to improved coverage of HIV and effective use of mass media

Target audiences: National media, CSOs, journalists

Primary approach: Media coverage

Description of intervention: The PPF sought to build the capacity of civil society professionals in Pakistan to work effectively with mass media in reducing HIV-related stigma and discrimination. The PPF organized five three-day training workshops on "Working with the Media" for CSOs in the cities of Abbottabad, Karachi, Lahore, and Quetta, and 119 civil society professionals participated in the training. The workshops for CSOs included NGOs working with groups at high risk for HIV, NGOs working with adolescents, and NGOs involved in general awareness-raising activities. The purpose of the workshops was to train NGO personnel how to cooperate with the media on their activities. Workshops included a panel discussion with experienced journalists from both the print and electronic media and taught participants to develop press releases and letters to the editor.

The PPF also sought to raise awareness of journalists and develop their capacity and writing skills for news reporting and feature writing on issues related to HIV and stigma and discrimination. The PPF organized five three-day awareness-raising workshops for local journalists in the cities of Karachi, Multan, Nathia Gali, and Sukkur. The workshops included (a) expert presentations to improve participants' knowledge of various aspects of HIV, (b) sessions on ethical issues and media guidelines for reporting on HIV, (c) discussions of what constitutes stigma and discrimination broadly with practical exercises depicting stigma through pictures and the participants' own experience of stigma, and (d) discussions with HIV-positive people about their actual experiences of stigma and discrimination. The workshops focused in parallel on building skills in news and feature writing.

Implementation, Results, and Challenges

Measurement strategies: All training participants were asked to take pre- and postknowledge tests and to fill out evaluation forms after each activity.

In pre- and posttests designed for journalists, questions assessed knowledge of the abbreviations related to HIV and AIDS, the prevalence of HIV in the world and in Pakistan, misused terms associated with HIV and AIDS, the general behavior of the public toward people living with HIV, and information about prevention. Questions in the pre- and posttests designed for NGO participants assessed knowledge of media (for example, the meaning of terms such as *intro, embargo, deadline, caption, news sense, press conference, interview, media plan,* and *follow-up*). Each questionnaire had 15 questions. For the journalists, the average pretest score was 4.6, and the average posttest score was 12.1; for the NGO participants, the average pretest score was 2.6, and the average posttest score was 13.7.

Results, key findings, and lessons: The PPF developed the capacity of 119 civil society professionals and 104 journalists in the training workshops.

As part of the workshops, each of the 104 journalist participants was to complete a feature article on HIV-related stigma and discrimination over the three-day period of the forum, starting with the outline at the end of the first day and continuing with discussion and finalization of the article by the end of the workshop. From the workshops, the journalists produced 107 feature articles, and the CSO representatives produced 187 press releases and letters to the editor in addition to 18 newsletters on issues related to HIV. The PPF obtained 31 published clippings of feature articles written by participants and 43 published stories about the events organized under the program. The PPF estimates the total number of published stories was at least twice the number of clippings received.

Overall, project successes included improved knowledge as a result of the workshop, an increase in the number of articles on HIV featured in local newspapers, and improved skills of NGO personnel in interacting and engaging with the media on HIV-related issues.

Challenges and unforeseen outcomes: Challenges identified by the PPF included managing open discussions with very conservative religious participants, who often raised objections to the content. Able resource persons who were also well versed in religious teachings and could use these teachings to support some key points were used to manage these challenges.

Because so little had been written about HIV in Pakistan, the PPF had difficulty initially identifying journalists who had experience writing about these issues. The PPF researched English and Urdu newspapers to look for journalists who had written news items, articles, or features on HIV. It was eventually able to identify and bring 104 journalists and reporters working for local newspapers across all provinces as well as the national papers to participate in the workshops.

Additional Information
Program references, media coverage, and materials developed: A list of the following materials developed is available on request:

- 31 published articles
- 47 unpublished articles
- 58 letters to the editor
- 55 press releases.

Contact information: Owais Aslam Ali, ppf@pakistanpressfoundation.org; aidsnewsdigest@pakistanpressfoundation.org

Additional funding, replication, or scale-up opportunities or new partnerships resulting from the project: The PPF worked closely with local representatives of the Joint United Nations Programme on HIV/AIDS (UNAIDS), which was very impressed by the quality of training. The UNAIDS country representative visited the PPF in December 2009 and expressed interest in working with the PPF to develop a training program for journalists on raising awareness of HIV and AIDS.

CHAPTER 17

Sri Lanka

Alliance Lanka

Project title: Our Health: Empowering Communities to Normalize HIV

Implementing organizations: Alliance Lanka and partner organizations: Community Strength for Development Foundation (Gampaha district), SERVE (Colombo), and the Wasone Foundation (Kurunegala)

Location: Kadawatha, Katunayake, Kelaniya, Peliyagoda, Ragama, and Wattala in Gampaha district; Moratuwa, Mt. Lavinia, and Ratmalana in Colombo district; Kurunegala, Mallawapitiya, and Maspotha in Kurunegala district

Background

Program goals: To improve awareness, education, and services on HIV in a nonthreatening environment and to facilitate voluntary counseling and referral for testing

Target audience: General population

Primary approach: Outreach

Description of intervention: The project involved four local nongovernmental organizations in efforts to provide training, advocacy, and voluntary counseling and testing (VCT) referrals to men and women living with HIV and AIDS across three districts in Sri Lanka. The four coordinating agencies developed a training curriculum for HIV-positive individuals on healthy living, and training was held in a local hospital serving HIV-positive patients (51 were trained). Project staff members were trained to provide follow-up every two months for training participants. A second training was developed on business planning and management for HIV-positive individuals and their families.

In addition, the project identified 48 locations for setting up furnished summer huts as roadside stands to provide information services. Visitors who came to the roadside stand were able to complete a questionnaire. Complementing the roadside stands were three people's centers. These centers were furnished spaces staffed by project facilitators who provided referrals and information about VCT and treatment for sexually transmitted infections. Counseling services were provided at the centers, and each center had recreational facilities. Other programs at the centers included education sessions on HIV and sexually transmitted infections, with some resource support from a local clinic, resource support on HIV-positive living from HIV-positive individuals, nutrition support from a nutritionist, and programs on domestic violence and family relationships provided by Alliance Lanka staff.

Each center had a telephone for those who preferred to call for assistance rather than appear in person. Contact information for the centers was provided at all of the roadside stands, and visitors to the roadside stands were encouraged to access more services through the centers.

Condoms from the National Sexually Transmitted Disease and AIDS Control Programme were distributed free of charge at the stands and centers. In addition, condom demonstrations and informational materials and posters were provided at the stands and the centers. An advocacy CD (compact disc) was also distributed through the centers.

Implementation, Results, and Challenges

Measurement strategies: Logbooks were kept of visitors to the roadside stands and the services provided at the stands and people's centers. People attending the 48 roadside stands completed 12,321 surveys.

Results, key findings, and lessons: Overall, 85 referrals to clinics for sexually transmitted infections and other counseling centers were made at the roadside stands, and 48 were made at the people's centers. The project's communication messages led 116 people to seek HIV testing at the centers. Project staff members felt the location of the stands and centers along with outreach activities encouraged community engagement and facilitated visits for information, advice, and services. The acceptability of this format for providing information on HIV and stigma is attested to by the requests Alliance Lanka received from other districts to conduct roadside stands in their districts. Project staff members felt that playing catchy music at the roadside stands evoked curiosity among the general public and drew people to seek information. Displaying the hotline numbers at the roadside stands also appeared to be important, because it resulted in many private phone calls from people who wished to obtain assistance in a confidential manner. Both project staff members and hotline users viewed the telephone hotline as a successful strategy for involving individuals who might otherwise be unwilling to seek counseling and referral for HIV testing and support. Some people who initially called on the hotline eventually came in person to receive HIV testing, counseling, and support. As a result of the business planning training, one HIV-positive participant received financial support to purchase a machine to cut coconut husk chips, and two others will reorient or expand their businesses with support from Alliance Lanka.

Over the course of the project, visitors to the roadside stands completed more than 12,000 questionnaires. Survey results indicated that general awareness of HIV was high; however, in-depth information about the modes of HIV transmission and prevention methods was fairly low. In addition, stigmatizing attitudes were quite prevalent among roadside stand visitors. For example, 42 percent of respondents believed that HIV is punishment for bad behavior, and 80 percent believed that people with HIV are promiscuous. Shame was also quite high, with 58 percent stating they would be ashamed if they were infected with HIV and 54 percent stating that people with HIV should be ashamed of themselves. These findings demonstrate that the general population in the intervention communities needs additional efforts to increase knowledge and awareness of HIV and to decrease stigma.

Challenges and unforeseen outcomes: Local security personnel at times objected to the activities at the roadside stands. This issue was resolved by engaging security personnel in friendly discussions and by obtaining approval documents.

Additional Information

Program references, media coverage, and materials developed: An advocacy CD featuring messages of HIV-positive living was produced with four people living with HIV and AIDS and was distributed through the people's centers.

Contact information: Swarna Kodagoda, swarna.kodagoda@gmail.com

Additional funding, replication, or scale-up opportunities or new partnerships resulting from the project: The National Tuberculosis Control Program requested that its activities be linked with the Alliance Lanka people's centers. This issue will be taken up in the Round 10 proposal to the Global Fund to Fight AIDS, Tuberculosis and Malaria.

Lanka+

Project title: Reducing Stigma and Discrimination Faced by People Living with and Affected by HIV/AIDS through Advocacy for Employment

Implementing organizations: Lanka+, International Labour Organization HIV/AIDS workplace program, International Labour Organization Start and Improve Your Business program, Sarvodaya Economic Enterprise Development Services (SEEDS) Guarantee Limited

Location: Obeysekerepura, Rajagiriya, and Waishakya Mawatha

Background

Program goals: To empower and reduce self-stigma among Lanka+ members through skills training, advocacy for employment, and income-generating activities

Target audiences: People living with HIV, general population

Primary approach: Employment

Description of intervention: At the onset of the project, Lanka+ conducted a market survey assessment to test the marketability of products, identify useful skills training, and guide its livelihood and income-generating project into a sustainable program with a strong business case.

To ensure that the program had a strong stigma reduction focus, the project selected participants on the basis of need, income, and skills and conducted a baseline assessment of attitudes and perceptions related to self-stigma. The project aimed to reduce self-stigma among 21 people living with HIV through training in business and marketing skills, as well as technical skills.

The training program for technical skills development (including candle making and screen printing, among other skills) was completed by 46 Lanka+ members. Twenty-one people living with HIV received financial support for implementing small-scale enterprises, and a revolving

loan fund was set up. The project developed a Web site (http://www
.lankaplus.org) for social marketing as part of the income-generating program. The Web site is in the process of being translated into local languages for the main target audiences. Products are currently being
marketed individually and through Lanka+. The project had the assistance of 30 undergraduate sociology students from the University of
Colombo in developing an awareness-raising campaign and product
launch organized for World AIDS Day 2009. They helped produce a
documentary of the project, as well as a brochure, posters, and t-shirts.

Implementation, Results, and Challenges
Measurement strategy: Marketing assessment survey

Results, key findings, and lessons: The main successes of the project were
(a) developing a training program for building technical skills, such as
business management, candle making and packaging, and screen printing; (b) training 20 women in a pilot marketing project; and (c) launch-
ing the Web site for social marketing purposes. As a result of the
project, the participants' self-confidence has increased, and they continue to apply management skills they learned from the training to their
business ventures.

Challenges and unforeseen outcomes: At the onset of the project, many of
the Lanka+ members were not open about their HIV status, had low self-
esteem, and had a high degree of self-stigma. In addition, many were living in poverty. Also challenging was the initial lack of confidence among
the Lanka+ members that their products would be accepted on the market. The project addressed this concern by recruiting an experienced project officer and holding meetings with Lanka+ members to explain the
potential benefits of the project.

Additional Information
Program references, media coverage, and materials developed:

- A Web site, http://www.lankaplus.org
- A documentary of the project
- Brochures, posters, and t-shirts

Contact information: Priyanthi Kumari, slplusnet@gmail.com

*Additional funding, replication, or scale-up opportunities or new partnerships
resulting from the project:* Additional funding was received from SEEDS.

South Asia Region Development Marketplace Summary Table

Grantee name, project title, and contact information	Target audiences	Primary program approaches	Key outputs	Monitoring and evaluation mechanisms[a]		
				Formative research	Program monitoring	Evaluation
AFGHANISTAN						
Afghan Family Guidance Association (AFGA) HIV and AIDS Stigma and Discrimination Reduction through Raising Awareness in Kabul City, Afghanistan Naimatullah Akbari, nakbari@afga.org.af	• Health workers • Prisoners • Prison staff members • Religious leaders • Youth • Media	• Training-of-trainers (TOT) program • Information, education, and communication (IEC) materials • Media coverage • Peer education	• Distributed 5,000 copies of poster on HIV and AIDS stigma and discrimination • Translated HIV and AIDS stigma and discrimination training toolkits into local languages • Trained 60 AFGA service providers, 25 medical and 91 nonmedical workers at prison centers, 28 prison peer educators, 13 AFGA youth peer educators, and 60 media representatives on HIV and AIDS stigma reduction • Trained 3 senior religious members who then trained about 75 junior religious leaders in Kabul		√	√

Organization/Program	Target audience	Type	Achievements		
Afghan Help and Training Program (AHTP) Tackling HIV and AIDS Stigma and Discrimination: From Insight to Action Amanullah Momand, dramanullah_momand@yahoo.com	Religious leaders: mullahs, mawlawies, mosque congregations	• TOT • IEC materials	• Produced new television (TV) announcements on HIV and AIDS stigma and discrimination, which were broadcast 3 times during December 2009 • Conveyed messages on HIV and AIDS and related stigma to more than 45,000 people in 5 districts of Jalalabad and distributed 6,000 posters and 60,000 leaflets • Completed TOT for 10 senior mawlawies and trained 300 mullahs as well as 30 members of the youth association	√	√
Concern Worldwide Addressing HIV and AIDS Related Stigma and Discrimination in Afghanistan Fiona McLysaght, fionamcly@yahoo.ie	• Health professionals • Mullahs • Teachers • Prison officers • Community leaders • Police officers • People living with HIV	Film	• Developed 6 films in Pashto and Dari • Assessed the knowledge of the participants in each course before and after showing the films and subsequently providing training on HIV and AIDS • Trained 400 individuals from 6 disparate groups on HIV and AIDS	√	√

(continued)

South Asia Region Development Marketplace Summary Table (*continued*)

Grantee name, project title, and contact information	Target audiences	Primary program approaches	Key outputs	Monitoring and evaluation mechanisms[a]		
				Formative research	Program monitoring	Evaluation
BANGLADESH						
Drik Picture Library Mainstreaming the Fringe Jeevani Fernando, jeevani @drik.net	• Role models • Activists • Media • Teachers • Members of the public	Media campaign (online)	• Conducted expert meeting of media stakeholders on training needs identification • Conducted training on online Web-video production for the media • Conducted roundtable talk shows • Collected oral testimonies for the Internet	√		
Job Opportunity and Business Support (JOBS)–Bangladesh Economic Rehabilitation of Intravenous Drug Users Elli Takagaki, elli@jobs-ict.com; info@jobs-group.org	• Public community • Injecting drug users (IDUs)	• Advocacy campaign • Employment services	• Trained 24 graduates from rehabilitation centers and established most as ambassadors in their communities • Created a sustainable production line of "red mannequins" in which profits are reinvested to hire more former IDUs		√	√

Project	Target group	Activities	Outcomes		
			• Showcased the red mannequins in 26 locations for awareness and advocacy purposes and gave presentations at 5 locations	√	
Nari Unnayan Shakti (Women's Power for Development) Reduction of Stigma and Discrimination on HIV/AIDS through Media Sensitization and Reporting in Bangladesh Afroja Parvin, nusbdwomen @yahoo.com	• Journalists • Members of the public	Media campaign	• Conducted training for 137 journalists on stigma reduction and oriented 288 journalists on sexually transmitted infection (STI) and AIDS prevention • Developed 130 articles and published 78 • Reprinted 1,500 copies of "AIDS Questions and Answers" and distributed 1,100 copies to journalists		
INDIA					
Ashodaya Samithi Addressing Stigma and Discrimination towards HIV+ Sex Workers and Sex Workers in General through Entrepreneurship Akram Pasha, ashodayasamithi @yahoo.co.in	Sex workers	• Advocacy campaign • Employment services	• Sensitized 65 health personnel, assisted 725 sex workers at the health facility, and created better health care access for 1,135 sex workers • Reduced violence from the police experienced by sex workers during the project period	√	√

(continued)

South Asia Region Development Marketplace Summary Table *(continued)*

Grantee name, project title, and contact information	Target audiences	Primary program approaches	Key outputs	Monitoring and evaluation mechanisms[a]		
				Formative research	Program monitoring	Evaluation
Development Initiative Fighting Discrimination amongst the Population Suffering Most from the Prejudices Attached to HIV/AIDS Sanjay Kumar, sanjay @developmentinitiative.org; kjsanjay@gmail.com	Members of the public	• Theater • Media (radio)	• Conducted 23 meetings or trainings for police personnel, conductors, and drivers, which social champions addressed • Trained 1,800 sex workers on issues involving stigma and discrimination, resulting in increased recognition and reporting of incidents of discrimination by sex workers • Increased restaurant's consumer base to serving 450–500 people daily • Trained 25 people working around the railway station in street theater, who put on 140 street theater performances • Formed a folk ballad group and put on 50 folk dance performances • Produced a 52-episode radio series for the National AIDS Coordinating Organisation		√	

	Target audience	Medium	Outputs		
ISTV Network Fighting Discrimination through Awareness: Game Show Yumnam Rupachandra Singh, yumnamrupa@gmail.com	Members of the public	Game show	• Aired 68 episodes across 4 districts to an estimated half million viewers • Recorded and aired 5 special episodes involving only individuals living with HIV and AIDS • Of viewers, 90% felt the game show was educational, and 94% felt the game show would help reduce stigma and discrimination.	√	√
Lotus Integrated AIDS Awareness Sangam Advocacy by Cultural Teams (ACT) N. Muthukumar, lotus_sangam @yahoo.co.in	• Village panchayat leaders • Community members	Theater	• Completed 75 village performances by ACT team • Completed 20 end-line interviews among panchayat leaders • Conducted 4 focus group discussions among village men who have sex with men (MSM) • Increased knowledge and acceptance of the MSM community by panchayats as an immediate outcome of performances	√	√

(continued)

South Asia Region Development Marketplace Summary Table *(continued)*

Grantee name, project title, and contact information	Target audiences	Primary program approaches	Key outputs	Monitoring and evaluation mechanisms[a] Formative research	Program monitoring	Evaluation
			• Helped MSM who participated in the ACT project to realize skills and potential many did not know they possessed • Identified new and hidden MSM through performances and linked them to services • Engaged and raised community awareness with performances (some drawing audiences upward of 300) • Received media attention			
Nalandaway Foundation Nalandaway Children Media Project Sriram Ayer, sriram@nalandaway.org	Members of the public	Film	• Trained 30 children in a 10-day participatory workshop in creative thinking, drama, photography, music, storytelling, and filmmaking	√		
Sai Paranjpye Films Qisse (Episodes) Sai Paranjpye, saiparanjpye@gmail.com	• Marginalized groups • Sex workers • IDUs • Organizations working with these groups	Film	• Researched and produced 2 films • Showed *Suee* at the International Conference on AIDS in Asia and the Pacific		√	

Organization	Target audience	Services	Achievements	✓
	• Members of the public		• *Suee* acquired by several organizations for screening among their members	✓
Saral Food and Catering Services for PLHA Hemalee Leuva, hemalee @ramanagroup.org	• Members of the public • People living with HIV	Employment services	• Developed terms of reference and business model for food procurement, production, and distribution services • Formed links with 5 institutions for training and food service delivery • Formed the Aadhar Mahila Trust to facilitate involvement in commercial activities and provide a platform for women living with HIV to gain confidence and sustainable livelihood	
Society for Positive Atmosphere and Related Support to HIV/AIDS (SPARSHA) Art and Testimonial: A Unique Community-Based Approach to Reduce HIV/AIDS Stigma in Villages of West Bengal Samiran Panda, dr.samiran _panda@rediffmail.com	• Members of the public • People living with HIV	• Community engagement • Solidarity between people living with HIV and those not infected with HIV • Traditional music and dance • Outreach	• Measured changes in attitude in community after first pilot intervention, and saw an increase in proportion of people disagreeing with 4 stigmatizing statements • Held 3 performances by Baul singers, once a week over a 3-week period in 4 intervention sites	✓

(continued)

South Asia Region Development Marketplace Summary Table *(continued)*

Grantee name, project title, and contact information	Target audiences	Primary program approaches	Key outputs	Monitoring and evaluation mechanisms[a]		
				Formative research	Program monitoring	Evaluation
Swathi Mahila Sangha Spoorthi: Community Action against Stigma and Discrimination: Project Baduku Pushpa Latha. R, sms-pragati @airtelmail.in	• Female sex workers • Female sex workers living with HIV	• Awareness training • Advocacy campaign	• Trained 384 female sex workers living with HIV through one-on-one training, events, and support groups • Oriented 450 HIV project staff members on stigma and discrimination and involved them in all major stigma reduction campaigns • Led 3 support group meetings for 35–50 members each, conducted in different parts of Bangalore every month on fixed dates • Received media exposure through more than 20 articles published in many Kannada and English newspapers and local TV channel telecast on HIV and women in sex work	√	√	

Program / Contact	Target audience	Approach	Activities and outcomes			
(continued from previous entry)			• Developed a pictorial community monitoring tool on stigma assessment and did 1 round of study with 166 female sex workers living with HIV to assess the level of internal and external stigma	√	√	√
The Communication Hub (TCH) Celebrating Those Who Care: A Radio Program by Positive Journalists Sonalini Mirchandani, sonalini @thecommunicationhub.com	• General population • People living with HIV	Media (radio)	• Produced 13 radio episodes • Trained 10 people living with HIV as radio journalists • Conducted 4 focus group discussions and 6 interviews after a pretest of 4 episodes • Conducted postproject survey of 7 journalists who were living with AIDS and 3 project team members			
Voluntary Health Association of Tripura (VHAT) Integrated Communication Strategy for Tackling HIV and AIDS Stigma and Discrimination in Tripura Sreelekha Ray, vha_tripura @rediffmail.com	• Religious leaders • Panchayat members • Media • Members of the defense force (Border Security Force) • Members of the public • People living with HIV	• Awareness training • IEC materials • Media coverage	• Conducted 10 training sessions for 583 participants, including 62 media personnel • Disseminated 500 copies of a booklet on HIV and STIs • Documented 10 cases of stigma and discrimination, provided support, and supplied legal support to 1 case • Received media coverage of program activities		√	

(continued)

South Asia Region Development Marketplace Summary Table *(continued)*

Grantee name, project title, and contact information	Target audiences	Primary program approaches	Key outputs	Monitoring and evaluation mechanisms[a]		
				Formative research	Program monitoring	Evaluation
We Care Social Service Society Promotion of Community Discussion and Debate Using Traditional Folk Media Known as *Therukoothu* (Street Drama) A. Antony Samy, wecareindia @gmail.com	• Members of the public • People living with HIV	Traditional theater	• Trained 5 people living with HIV to perform and participate in community theater and discussions • Performed HIV-related dramas with follow-on discussion for 10 villages, 3 times per village • Increased audience participation • Facilitated access to services available through nongovernmental organizations and government hospitals for people living with HIV in the villages where performances were held • Conducted 20 focus group discussions and 7 key informant interviews with women's self-help groups, youth, village leaders, and village elders	√	√	√

NEPAL

Organization	Target audience	Activity	Outcomes
Federation of Sexual and Gender Minorities Nepal (FSGMN) Beauty and Brains in Action to Tackle HIV/AIDS Stigma and Discrimination Sunil Babu Pant, beauty.and.brain2008 @gmail.com Subash Pokharel, bluediamondsociety @yahoo.com	• Members of the public • MSM • Transgender community	• Beauty pageant • Advocacy campaign (ambassadorship of winners)	• Declared and appointed 5 winners as regional HIV ambassadors; declared 1 contestant as national ambassador • Received attendance of approximately 1,500 audience members at 6 pageants • Received coverage in mainstream print media and electronic media and Web space for MSM or transgender groups to cover topics on HIV and AIDS and human rights • Through ambassadors and other participants, convinced new donors to bring prevention programs on HIV for MSM and transgender individuals to 14 districts in Nepal

√

(continued)

South Asia Region Development Marketplace Summary Table (continued)

Grantee name, project title, and contact information	Target audiences	Primary program approaches	Key outputs	Monitoring and evaluation mechanisms[a]		
				Formative research	Program monitoring	Evaluation
Himalayan Association against STI-AIDS (HASTI-AIDS) Addressing HIV and AIDS Related Stigma and Discrimination through Social, Economic, and Institutional Interventions in Achham District Nirmal Kumar Bista, hastiaids@mcmail.com.np; nkbista@yahoo.com	• General population • People living with HIV • Migrants and their families • Health workers • Teachers • Students • Journalists • Volunteers • Opinion leaders	• Awareness trainings • Street drama • Media (radio) • Peer educators	• Completed 10 focus group discussions with people living with HIV, teachers, migrants and their spouses, and health care providers • Held 2 meetings with income-generating programs to better involve people living with HIV • Assessed the actions of peer educators during 3 meetings • Collaborated with a local drama group to perform 9 street dramas in local dialects at important local festivals • Held an orientation workshop with the District AIDS Coordination Committee to regularly review progress in stigma and discrimination reduction of participating organizations • Participated in finalization of scripts for radio learning programs		√	√

Organization/Project	Target audience	Activities	Results	
National NGOs Network Group against AIDS–Nepal (Nangan) Creating PLHA-Friendly Hospitals: Improving the Hospital Environment for HIV-Positive Clients in Nepalese Regional Hospitals Usha Jha, ushajha05@yahoo.com	• Health workers • HIV-positive patients	• TOT • IEC materials	• Implemented client satisfaction survey ($n = 204$) in each hospital at 3 points during November and June 2009 (baseline, midline, and end line) • Conducted TOT with 66 health workers across 3 hospitals • Formed client satisfaction committees at each hospital and formed a working task team to review existing policies and practices in consultation with policy makers	√
PAKISTAN				
Integrated Health Services (IHS) Advocacy Campaign to Reduce AIDS Stigma by Creating "HIV Forums" at Colleges in Islamabad Muhammad Asim Mahmood Khan, asim@ihspakistan.com; ihspakistan@hotmail.com	University and college students 17–25 years of age	Organization of youth forums	At 5 universities, 462 students completed the preintervention knowledge, attitudes, and practices to inform development of youth forums and content of educational materials and presentation.	√

(continued)

South Asia Region Development Marketplace Summary Table *(continued)*

Grantee name, project title, and contact information	Target audiences	Primary program approaches	Key outputs	Monitoring and evaluation mechanisms[a]		
				Formative research	Program monitoring	Evaluation
New Light AIDS Control Society (NLACS) Reducing Stigma to Improve Uptake for Antiretroviral Treatment and Community Home-Based Care among People Living with HIV and AIDS, Men Who Have Sex with Men, and Individuals from the Transgender Community Asher Bhatti; newlightaids @gmail.com	• MSM • People living with HIV • Transgender individuals	TOT	• Strengthened ties with local hospitals and voluntary counseling and testing centers, both public and private, resulting in expansion of NLACS referral system to 36 villages, adding 6 new facilities to the referral system • Conducted a seminar with 23 media personnel who then made commitments to reduce stigma and discrimination through more accurate reporting in print and broadcast media and agreed to receive news stories and information from NLACS for dissemination • Trained 24 health workers in basic information about MSM and transgender individuals		√	√

Organization / Project	Target groups	Intervention type	Results			
Pakistan Press Foundation (PPF) Capacity Development of Media and Civil Society Organizations to Improve Coverage of HIV/AIDS Owais Aslam Ali ppf @pakistanpressfoundation .org; aidsnewsdigest @pakistanpressfoundation.org	• National media • Civil society organizations • Journalists	Media	• Developed the capacity of 119 civil society professions and 104 journalists in training workshops • Produced 107 feature articles and 187 press releases and letters to the editor, in addition to 18 newsletters on issues related to HIV, through journalist participants in workshops • Obtained 31 published clippings of feature articles written by participants and 43 published stories about the events organized under the program • Increased knowledge about HIV and AIDS and the proper way to discuss the topic among training participants		√	√
SRI LANKA *Alliance Lanka* Our Health: Empowering Communities to Normalize HIV Swarna Kodagoda, swarna .kodagoda@gmail.com	• People living with HIV • Members of the public	• IEC materials • Training	• Established 48 roadside stands to provide information and referral to support centers • Obtained completed questionnaires about HIV and AIDS knowledge from 12,276 of 12,540 visitors to roadside stands	√	√	

(continued)

South Asia Region Development Marketplace Summary Table (continued)

Grantee name, project title, and contact information	Target audiences	Primary program approaches	Key outputs	Monitoring and evaluation mechanisms[a]		
				Formative research	Program monitoring	Evaluation
			• Established 3 support centers that continue to function after the project grant period • Held training for people living with HIV on positive living and business skills			
Lanka+ Reducing Stigma and Discrimination Faced by People Living with and Affected by HIV/AIDS through Advocacy for Employment Priyanthi Kumari, slplusnet @gmail.com	• People living with HIV • Members of the public	Employment services	• Trained 46 members in technical skills • Launched a social marketing Web site in English and local languages • Conducted rapid assessment of program beneficiaries • Issued 21 loans to beneficiaries to establish small enterprises		√	

Source: Authors.

a. *Formative research* is collecting data through baseline surveys, baseline focus group discussions, and baseline key informant interviews. *Program monitoring* is collecting data on the number of tasks completed. *Evaluation* is collecting data through pre- and posttraining surveys, end-line surveys, end-line focus group discussions, and end-line key informant interviews.

Index

Boxes, notes, and tables are indicated by b, n, and t following the page numbers.

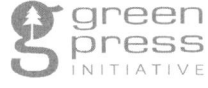